OTHER MONOGRAPHS IN THE SERIES
MAJOR PROBLEMS IN PATHOLOGY

Benjamin Wittels, M.D.
Department of Pathology
Duke University School of Medicine
Durham, North Carolina

Surgical Pathology
of
Bone Marrow — *Core Biopsy Diagnosis*

Volume 17 in the Series
MAJOR PROBLEMS IN PATHOLOGY

JAMES L. BENNINGTON, M.D., *Consulting Editor*
Chairman, Department of Pathology
Children's Hospital of San Francisco
San Francisco, California

W. B. SAUNDERS COMPANY

Philadelphia, London, Toronto, Mexico City, Rio de Janeiro, Sydney, Tokyo, Hong Kong

W. B. Saunders Company: West Washington Square
                          Philadelphia, PA   19105

Library of Congress Cataloging in Publication Data

Wittels, Benjamin.

Surgical Pathology of Bone Marrow.

(Major problems in pathology; v. 17)

1. Marrow—Diseases—Diagnosis.   2. Marrow—Biopsy.
3. Diagnosis, Cytologic.   I. Bennington, James L.
(James Lynne), 1935–   II. Title. [DNLM: 1. Bone
Marrow Diseases—pathology.   2. Bone Marrow Examination.   3. Lymphatic Diseases—pathology. W1 MA492X
v.17/WH 380 W828b]

RC645.7.W57 1985   616.4'10758   84–23539

ISBN 0–7216–1434–5

Surgical Pathology of Bone Marrow   ISBN 0–7216–1434–5

Last digit is the print number: 9   8   7   6   5   4   3   2

Preface

Core biopsy of the bone marrow has become an accepted, if not an indispensable, procedure in evaluating the hematologic status of a patient. For informational content, the microscopic section of the core has all but replaced that of the aspirated marrow particle and in many respects ranks abreast or exceeds the standard marrow particle smear. The simplicity and safety of the core biopsy technique have promoted its wide use, but its ultimate value rests on the capability of the microscopist interpreting the section. From a practical viewpoint, this monograph seeks to enhance the diagnostic ability of those who practice morphologic hematology. From a broader perspective, the monograph attempts to conceptualize individual diseases or groups of diseases in order to improve the understanding of the pathogenesis of their manifestations. The aim of both approaches is better treatment of the patient. To the extent that these goals are achieved, the monograph will have succeeded in its intended purpose.

BENJAMIN WITTELS, M.D.

Acknowledgment

Several members of the Pathology Department were supportive in the preparation of this monograph. They included Mr. Phillip Pickett, head of the histology laboratory, and his very able staff; Mr. William Boyarsky, formerly head of the photography laboratory; Miss Susan Reeves, current head of the photography laboratory; and Mrs. Sara Lyon and Mrs. Diane Evans, secretaries, who with dedication and insistence on perfection were largely responsible for the processing of the text. I am also indebted to the many physicians attending the Hematology Clinic, Department of Medicine, Duke Hospital, whose careful clinical records of patients I reviewed. Two are worthy of special mention: Dr. Harold Silberman and Dr. Joseph Moore. Finally, to Mrs. Hana Geber, artist and sculptor, New York City, I owe an immeasurable debt of gratitude.

BENJAMIN WITTELS, M.D.

Contents

1

GENERAL STATEMENT

Twenty-five years have passed since the introduction of the bone marrow needle biopsy by McFarland and Dameshek.[1] The value of this innovation was quickly recognized, and its acceptance has become generalized. Within five years the experience at several clinics was reported, and the general diagnostic applicability and utility as well as the specific merits of the procedure were defined.[2] Improved instruments were developed. Currently in the United States the Jamshidi needle is preferred.[3] A critical and balanced evaluation presented after almost 20 years of experience with the marrow core biopsy concluded that the combination of the aspiration-smear preparation and the core section preparation was the most expeditious and fruitful approach for evaluation of the marrow status.[4]

The technique used to obtain the marrow core specimen has been described repeatedly. Descriptions are available in the original publications and in standard textbooks of hematology[2,5] and need no repetition here. Similarly, the standard procedures applied to prepare the histologic sections are in general use and are described in some of these sources as well as in texts on histologic technique.[6] At the Duke Hospital in Durham, North Carolina, marrow core specimens are fixed and decalcified simultaneously in Zenker's solution-glacial acetic acid (95/5: volume per volume, v:v) overnight. Sequential sections, 6 microns thick, are prepared from the paraffin-embedded tissue and stained by a hematoxylin-eosin procedure or with the Prussian blue staining procedure. Special staining procedures are limited to those useful for detection of microorganisms and to those proteins currently demonstrable by immunocytochemical methods applicable to tissue processed as described. To date, the demonstration of immunoglobulins, hemoglobin, myoglobin, keratin, prostatic acid phosphatase, and lysozyme has proved useful in analysis of marrow core specimens.[7] There is promise that additional monoclonal antibodies may become available for the identification of other specific substances, including surface receptors, antigens, and immunoglobulins that remain stable during the standard preparative procedures.[8,9] The laborious methods now available can thereby be avoided.

The reticulin and collagen stains are overvalued for the information gained when they are applied to marrow core specimens. The presence of reticulin is nonspecific, and the presence of collagen can be clearly visualized in the standard section stained with hematoxylin and eosin. Accordingly, those special stains serve no useful purpose in diagnostic hematology.

The source material upon which all descriptive statements and conclusions in this monograph are based and from which all microphotographs were obtained is the sum total of iliac crest marrow core biopsy specimens originating during the study and treatment of patients at the Duke Hospital. Approximately 1000 such biopsies are done each year. No autopsy material has been used. With few exceptions, all the photographs represent standard hematoxylin-eosin–stained sections. Aside from a single photograph of a section stained for reticulin, all the exceptions are representations demonstrating the potential value of the immunoperoxidase procedure.

The normal marrow as such is not discussed. From the specific features of each disease state, the normal state can generally be surmised. The marrow cellularity, that is, the hematopoietic cell density, in the iliac crest as a function of age is the subject of a useful publication that includes photographs that can serve as a frame of reference for this variable.[10] The qualitative characteristics of the several cell lineages in the normal marrow can be learned from standard texts on histology. Study of the prevailing cells in the hematological diseases as illustrated in the relevant photographs in this monograph accomplish the same result.

Those who seek photographs of cryostat, superthin, or electron microscopic preparations will be disappointed. These have been studiously avoided for several reasons: (1) The techniques are laborious and time-consuming and with the exceptions noted later add little useful information when applied to the marrow core specimen. The standard procedure routinely requires 24 to 48 hours and can be reduced to 12 hours if necessary. (2) Disease in the marrow is commonly focal rather than diffuse. These techniques seriously curtail the amount of tissue that can be examined. This limitation is especially relevant in the evaluation of lymphomas, metastatic carcinomas, and the postchemotherapy status of the marrow because the reliability of the biopsy in detecting disease is proportional to the quantity of tissue examined. (3) The great majority of cells in normal and pathological marrow can be identified in the standard microscopic section as readily as in preparations using these techniques and in some instances with greater assurance. This fact is especially evident in distinguishing blast leukemias from metastatic undifferentiated carcinomas. Currently these criticisms directed at the routine application of the special techniques to the marrow core biopsy specimen do not apply to the diagnosis of acute megakaryoblastic leukemia, to the identification of mast cells, and to the clonal evaluation of focal deposits of well-differentiated lymphocytes. These problems are discussed in the appropriate sections. The immunoperoxidase technique can be expected to remove these limitations in the near future.

The audience to which this monograph is primarily directed includes pathologists, hematologists, and oncologists, both trained and in training. Each section on specific groups of primary hematological diseases is prefaced by a general statement on the scope and theory of the diseases and the involved cells. Each disease is presented by means of an exposition complemented by microphotographs, frequently at several levels of magnification. The multistep enlargements are purposeful. The trained microscopist recognizes that decisive information is accrued at each level of magnification, and only the novice "leaps" to view the tissue at the highest magnification and goes astray among the intracellular organelles. The cliché that a good photograph is worth a thousand words remains valid in imparting information in diagnostic microscopy of the bone marrow. Viewing selected microphotographs through a hand lens can also enhance their value. Portions of the exposition and selected photographs on each disease are more useful than others to the trained specialist; the entire exposition and all photographs may serve the novice. For the latter, this monograph is meant to be used in conjunction with a general treatise on hematology. Specific references thereto are given with most expositions. For the same group, many "picture books" are available to show cells as they appear in standard smear preparations of peripheral blood and bone marrow. No repetition of the products of this technique of study is therefore deemed necessary here.

REFERENCES

1. McFarland, W., and Dameshek, W.: Biopsy of bone marrow with the Vim-Silverman needle. JAMA 166:1464–1466, 1958.
2. Ellis, L. D., Jensen, W. N., and Westerman, M. P.: Needle biopsy of bone and marrow. Arch Intern Med 114:213–221, 1964.
3. Jamshidi, K., and Swain, W.: Bone marrow biopsy with unaltered architecture. J Lab Clin Med 77:333–342, 1971.
4. Block, M.: Bone marrow examination. Arch Pathol Lab Med 100:454–456, 1976.
5. Williams, W. J.: Examination of the marrow. In Williams, W. J., Beutler, E., Erslev, A. J., and Lichtman, M. A. (eds.): Hematology. New York, McGraw-Hill, 1983, pp. 25–32.
6. Carson, F. L., Matthews, J. L., and Pickett, J. P.: Preparation of tissue for laboratory examination. In Race, G. J. (ed.): Laboratory Medicine. Chap. 22. New York, Harper & Row, 1975.
7. Pinkus, G. S.: Diagnostic immunocytochemistry of paraffin-embedded tissues. Human Pathol 13:411–415, 1982.
8. Warnke, R. A., Gatter, K. C., Falini, B., et al.: Diagnosis of human lymphoma with monoclonal anti-leukocyte antibodies. N Engl J Med 309:1275–1281, 1983.
9. Moir, D. J., Ghosh, A. K., Abdulaziz, Z., et al.: Immunoenzymatic staining of haematological samples with monoclonal antibodies. Br J Haematol 55:395–410, 1983.
10. Hartsock, R. J., Smith, E. B., and Petty, C. S.: Normal variations with aging of the amount of hematopoietic tissue in bone marrow from the anterior iliac crest. Am J Clin Pathol 43:326–331, 1965.

2

THE MYELOPROLIFERATIVE DISEASES

CONCEPT AND SCOPE

The gathering of the myeloproliferative diseases into a unitary group can be justified on the basis of the properties they share in common. Among these are the following: (1) All of the cells that participate in these leukemias normally reside and mature in the marrow. (2) For each of the chronic leukemias in the group examined to date, evidence has been obtained that irrespective of the prevailing lineage all three "myeloid" cell lines—the red cell, the granulocyte, and the megakaryocyte—are neoplastic.[1] In the acute leukemias, however, the lines involved may be more restricted so that only one may be neoplastic.[2] (3) In addition to the prevailing cell abnormality, each type of leukemia frequently exhibits quantitative and qualitative abnormalities in the other two "myeloid" lines, whether the latter are neoplastic or not. (4) In the chronic forms of these leukemias, all exhibit splenomegaly but little or no lymph node enlargement. (5) All frequently have hyperuricemia, elevated serum lactic acid dehydrogenase, and increased serum B_{12} levels.

Seven acute and six chronic leukemias are incorporated in this disease category. The acute forms are myeloblastic, myeloblastic with maturation, myelomonocytic, monocytic, promyelocytic, erythroblastic, and megakaryocytic; the chronic leukemias are chronic granulocytic leukemia, chronic myelomonocytic leukemia, chronic monocytic leukemia, polycythemia vera, essential thrombocythemia, and chronic primary myelofibrosis.

Except for the delineation of acute promyelocytic leukemia as a special type of leukemia and the recognition of acute megakaryocytic leukemia, the group essentially retains the membership initially conceived by Dameshek.[3]

In view of the multifactor common denominator characterizing these leukemias, there has been a pervasive tendency to consider them as a spectrum of overlapping diseases whose defining edges are frequently blurred. This notion has been reinforced by interpreting progressions in the diseases as transformations or conversions. This explanation, while intellectually satisfying, is becoming increasingly untenable as more basic information on the diseases becomes available. Three examples serve to emphasize this point: (1) Chronic granulocytic leukemia labeled by the Philadelphia chromosome does not convert to just another indistinguishable case of acute myeloblastic leukemia when it progresses to blast crisis. Instead, the cells retain their stigmatizing chromosomes but simply lose their maturational capability.[4] (2) Polycythemia vera does not convert to another disease, myelosclerosis with myeloid metaplasia, but merely develops reactive fibrosis probably consequent to the aberrant behavior of its neoplastic megakaryocytes.[5] (3) Chronic primary myelofibrosis in progressing to acute leukemia does not necessarily convert only or even most frequently to acute myeloblastic leukemia. It has been shown that neoplastic megakaryocytes can lose their ability to mature and escape into the circulation as megakaryoblasts to produce a megakaryoblastic leukemia.[6] In addition, recent studies have indicated that the same cell lineage has different and distinctive cytokinetic properties in both differentiation and maturation in the different myeloproliferative diseases.[7-9] Finally, available information indicates that in each of these leukemias the chromosomal abnormality, when present, is idiotypic.[10] Thus, while the diseases in this group may have phenotypic overlap, they retain genotypic individuality.

Currently, most perplexing problems involving interpretation of marrow core specimens in this group of diseases center on cases with features considered to be consistent with myelodysplasia, malignant myelosclerosis, or acute megakaryoblastic leukemia. Analysis of the relevant publications in conjunction with personal experience has led to the conclusion that malignant myelosclerosis is not a disease entity and that after expurgating blatantly misdiagnosed cases such as acute myeloblastic leukemia with collagen fibrosis the reported cases that remain are either myelodysplasia or acute megakaryoblastic leukemia. The basis for this conclusion is given in detail in the relevant sections and in the exposition Myelosclerosis with Myeloid Metaplasia: A Revised View.

Many publications have emphasized the presence of fibrosis, reticulin or collagen, or both, as being of paramount significance in the diagnosis and differential diagnosis of these diseases. Sufficient evidence is currently available to conclude that marrow fibrosis is neither neoplastic nor specific for any of these diseases, although it may have a functional role in producing the manifestations of the disease. This statement can be generalized to the dictum that a diagnosis of marrow fibrosis or myelofibrosis is etiologically meaningless and diagnostically nonspecific.

The sequence in which the diseases are presented in this chapter is conventional: the acute are followed by the chronic, and generally the more frequent precede the less common. The myelodysplasias are included here because cases progressing to leukemia usually develop a form belonging to this group. A discussion of the marrow of patients with treated leukemia concludes the chapter. Most experience in evaluating core biopsy specimens of chemically treated leukemia has been accrued with acute myeloblastic leukemia. There is no evidence, however, that the response to chemotherapy in other leukemias or lymphomas is significantly different.

1. Adamson, J. W., and Fialkow, P. J.: The pathogenesis of myeloproliferative syndromes. Br J Haematol 38:299–303, 1978.
2. Fialkow, P. J., Singer, J. W., Adamson, J. W., et al.: Acute nonlymphocytic leukemia. N Engl J Med 301:1–5, 1979.
3. Dameshek, W., and Gunz, F.: Leukemia. New York, Grune & Stratton, 1958, pp. 262–297.
4. Koeffler, H. P., and Gold, D. W.: Chronic myelogenous leukemia—new concepts. N Engl J Med 304:1201–1209, 1981.
5. Groopman, J. E.: The pathogenesis of myelofibrosis in myeloproliferative disorders. Ann Intern Med 92:857–858, 1980.
6. Efrati, P., Nir, E., Yaari, A., et al.: Myeloproliferative disorders terminating in acute micromegakaryoblastic leukemia. Br J Haematol 43:79–86, 1979.
7. Singer, J. W., Adamson, J. W., Arlin, Z. A., et al.: Chronic myelogenous leukemia. J Clin Invest 67:1593–1598, 1981.
8. Adamson, J. W., Singer, J. W., and Catalano, P.: Polycythemia vera. J Clin Invest 66:1363–1368, 1980.
9. Kornberg, A., Fibach, E., Treves, A., et al: Circulating erythroid progenitors in patients with "spent" polycythaemia vera and myelofibrosis with myeloid metaplasia. Br J Haematol 52:573–578, 1982.
10. Rowley, J. D.: Cytogenetic studies in hematologic disorders. *In* Hoffbrand, A. V. (ed.): Recent Advances in Haematology. Edinburgh, Churchill Livingstone, 1982, pp. 233–252.

ACUTE MYELOBLASTIC, MYELOMONOCYTIC, AND MONOCYTIC LEUKEMIAS

The acute leukemias known as myeloblastic, myelomonocytic, and monocytic, with or without limited degrees of maturation, are considered collectively because of congruities in many clinical, morphological, cytochemical, and chemoresponsive properties. A theoretical basis for their joint consideration is provided by a well-known differentiation and maturation scheme of hematopoietic cells.[1] Supported by much data, this scheme postulates that the relevant cells in these leukemias arise from the same progenitor cell, which can be channeled uniquely into either the myeloblastic or the monoblastic pathway. This concept would explain the mixed and fluctuating cell population in myelomonocytic leukemia as well as the pure myeloblastic and monoblastic proliferations. One of the classic controversies in hematology can thus be satisfactorily resolved.*

---

*Admittedly, a rationale for classifying the acute monocytic and myelomonocytic leukemias with the histiocytic proliferative diseases can also be developed.[1]

In the widely publicized *French-American-British (FAB) classification* of acute myeloid leukemias, these diseases are designated as M-1 (myeloblastic leukemia without maturation), M-2 (myeloblastic leukemia with maturation), M-4 (myelomonocytic leukemia), and M-5 (monocytic leukemia).[2, 3] They represent 10, 30, 37, and 9 per cent, respectively, of the *acute myeloid leukemias* or what are fashionably referred to as the *acute nonlymphoblastic leukemias*. A member of this group, promyelocytic leukemia, known as M-3 in the FAB classification, is treated separately because of its singular clinical and morphological characteristics. For similar reasons, erythroleukemia, designated as M-6 in the FAB classification, is also discussed in a separate section.

As in all forms of leukemia, the diagnosis in these acute leukemias depends ultimately on examination of both the blood and bone marrow.[4, 5] For this purpose the marrow core specimen is no less valuable than smear preparations of marrow aspirates. When there are no abnormal cells in the blood and aspiration of the marrow is nonproductive, the core specimen can yield the required diagnostic proof. The cytochemistry currently used in distinguishing the several acute leukemias is applicable primarily to smear preparations.[2–4] Special and laborious fixation, and embedding procedures must be used for their application to core specimens. The immunoperoxidase technique is rapidly removing this barrier, since tissue fixed and processed by standard methods can be used to demonstrate the presence of identifying enzymes and products.[6] It should be emphasized that although subclassification is commonly corroborated by use of the smear preparations with confirmatory cytochemistry or by immunological procedures, the diagnosis of acute leukemia can be made with a high degree of reliability from the standard hematoxylin-eosin–stained sections of the core biopsy specimen.

In the core biopsy specimen the marrow space as a rule is densely populated with hematopoietic cells. The most arresting feature is the striking impairment of maturation. In the extreme case this is manifested by a marrow solidly packed with only hematopoietic blast cells. In many cases numbers of promyelocytes are admixed with the blast cells, and in others more mature forms are also present. In an occasional case, fat cells predominate, and the blast cells and their progeny are restricted to the interstices. Various texts and monographs state that a minimum of 40 to 60 per cent of blast cells in the marrow population is required for a definitive diagnosis of acute leukemias. Recently, the FAB group has set the threshold at 30 per cent.[7]

Two forms of blast cells occur, separately or in varying mixtures in the M-1, M-2, and M-4 types: (1) those with round to oval nuclei, usually punctuated by an obvious nucleolus (Figs. 2–1A and B), and (2) those with irregularly dented, folded, or twisted nuclei in which the nucleolus is inconspicuous (Figs. 2–2A and B). In both forms the chromatin tends to be coarse or clumped. Importantly, moderate amounts of granular cytoplasm ring the nucleus. By contrast, the lymphoblast of the L-1 type has a round nucleus, finely dispersed chromatin, an obscure nucleolus, and cytoplasm that is barely visible. The marrow population is remarkably homogeneous in these cases. The L-2 type of lymphoblast, on the other hand, has an irregular, folded, or dented nucleus and thus apes the myeloblast with the irregular nucleus. In the lymphoblast, however, the chromatin is finely dispersed and the cytoplasm barely visible.

A subgroup of acute myelomonocytic leukemia has been identified in which quantitative and qualitative abnormalities of eosinophils complement the usual features of the disease in the marrow and occasionally in the blood.[8] A specific chromosomal defect occurs in these cases, which is inversion of chromosome 16. Recognition is important because better than average length of remission can be expected following chemotherapy.

In the far less common monocytic leukemia (M-5)[9, 10] the blast cells are distinctive in that many have abundant eosinophilic cytoplasm surrounding centrally or eccentrically placed nuclei (Fig. 2–3). The nuclei are large, round to oval, or reniform and commonly contain a visible nucleolus. Some of the larger and perhaps more mature cells have a distinct resemblance to histiocytes.

Megakaryocytes, when present, are usually structurally abnormal. This abnormality may take the form of hyperlobulation of the nucleus, giant nuclear lobes, eccentric crowding of the nuclear lobes, bizarre cell shape, and too much or too little cytoplasm (Fig. 2–4).

The representation of the erythroid lineage varies from none to as much as 25 per cent of the hematopoietic cells. In some cases early normoblasts are conspicuously numerous, and in others late forms prevail. Even

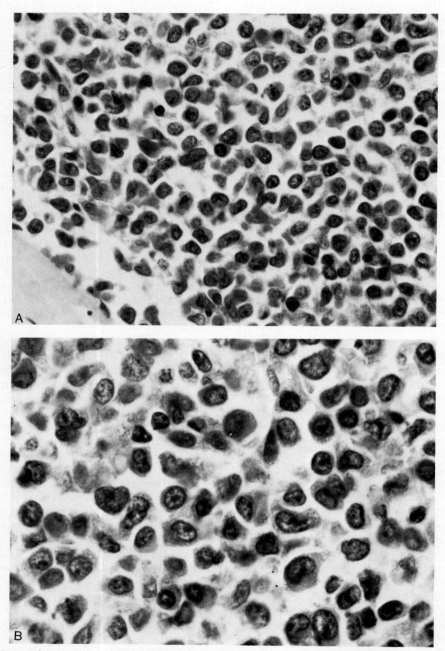

Figure 2–1. *A* and *B*. Acute myeloblastic leukemia in which most blast cells have a round to oval nucleus with an obvious nucleolus and contain a relatively abundant amount of cytoplasm. 680× and 1000×, hematoxylin and eosin stain (H&E).

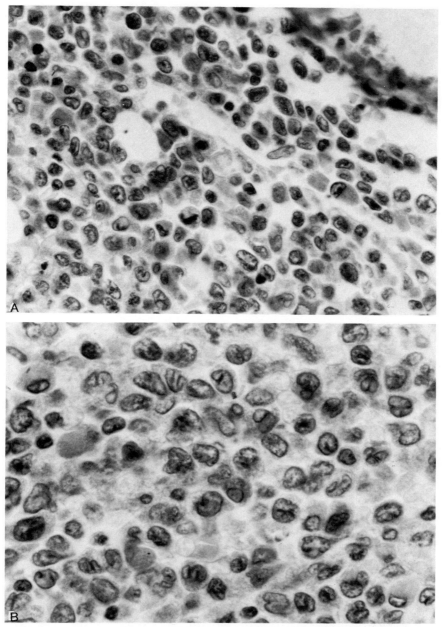

Figure 2–2. *A* and *B*. Acute myelomonocytic leukemia in which most blast cells have a highly irregular folded or indented nucleus. Nucleoli are inconspicuous if present. Most blast cells have relatively abundant cytoplasm. 680× and 1000×, H&E.

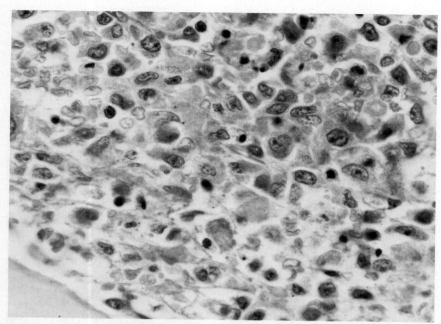

Figure 2–3. Acute monocytic leukemia in which the blast cells have a round to oval to reniform nucleus containing a small nucleus and dispersed chromatin. Large amounts of cytoplasm impart a histiocytic appearance to many cells. 680×, H&E.

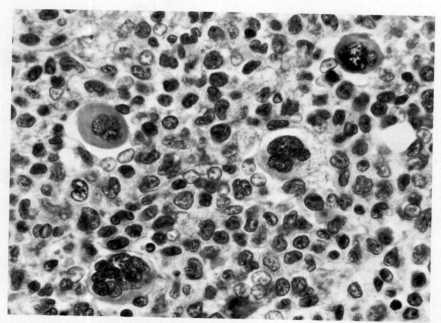

Figure 2–4. Acute myelomonocytic leukemia with a somewhat increased number of megakaryocytes. The megakaryocytes are distributed as singlets and have atypical nuclei, as indicated by hyper- and anisometric lobation. The leukemic blast cells possess the irregular, folded, or indented nucleus without a conspicuous nucleolus, which is the principal identifying feature of this type of leukemia. 680×, H&E.

prior to chemotherapy and in the presence of normal or high serum B_{12} and folate levels, the former may be indicative of defective maturation.

Differential diagnostic considerations are (1) acute lymphoblastic leukemia, (2) erythroleukemia, (3) large cell lymphoma, and (4) malignant histiocytosis. The features useful for distinguishing this group of acute leukemias from the acute lymphoblastic leukemias have been stated. The discrimination from erythroleukemia, which centers on the erythroblastic representation, is discussed in the section on erythroleukemia. The distinction from large cell lymphoma of the noncleaved type is on occasion problematic. Usually these large lymphocytes have such large nuclei with strikingly prominent nucleoli that there is no confusion with the myeloblast. Cases in which the diagnosis is questionable can be resolved by use of the immunoperoxidase method to demonstrate lysozyme activity in the myeloid group of leukemias. Cytochemical procedures applied to smear preparations can also be used. Finally, the differentiation of these acute leukemias, especially the monocytic form, from the rare disease malignant histiocytosis is possible on the basis of the heterogeneity of the cell population, which ranges from blast cells through monocytes to phagocytizing macrophages in the latter disease.[11]

REFERENCES

1. Cline, M. J., and Golde, D. W.: Controlling the production of blood cells. Blood 53:157–165, 1979.
2. Bennett, J. M., Catovsky, D., Daniel, M. T., et al.: Proposals for the classification of the acute leukemias. Br J Haematol 33:451–458, 1976.
3. Gralnick, H. R., Galton, D. A. G., Catovsky, D., et al.: Classification of acute leukemia. Ann Intern Med 87:740–753, 1977.
4. Henderson, E. S.: Acute leukemia. *In* Williams, W. J., Beutler, E., Erslev, A. J., and Lichtman, M. A. (eds.): Hematology. New York, McGraw-Hill, 1983, pp. 221–239.
5. Henderson, E. S.: Acute myelogenous leukemia. *In* Williams, W. J., Beutler, E., Erslev, A. J., and Lichtman, M. A. (eds.): Hematology. New York, McGraw-Hill, 1983, pp. 239–253.
6. Pinkus, G. S., and Said, J. W.: Profile of intracytoplasmic lysozyme in normal tissues, myeloproliferative disorders, hairy cell leukemia, and other pathologic processes: An immunoperoxidase study of paraffin sections and smears. Am J Pathol 89:351–366, 1977.
7. Bennett, J. M., Catovsky, D., Daniel, M. T., et al.: Proposals for the classification of the myelodysplastic syndromes. Br J Haematol 51:189–199, 1982.
8. LeBeau, M. M., Larson, R. A., Bitter, M. A., et al.: Association of an inversion of chromosome 16 with abnormal marrow eosinophils in acute myelomonocytic leukemia. N Engl J Med 309:630–636, 1983.
9. McKenna, R. W., Bloomfield, C. D., Dick, F., et al.: Acute monoblastic leukemia: Diagnosis and treatment of ten cases. Blood 46:481–494, 1975.
10. Shaw, M. T., and Nordquist, R. E.: Pure monocytic or histiomonocytic leukemia: A revised concept. Cancer 35:208–214, 1975.
11. Lampert, I. A., Catovsky, D., and Bergier, N.: Malignant histiocytosis: A clinico-pathological study of 12 cases. Br J Haematol 40:65–77, 1978.

ACUTE PROMYELOCYTIC LEUKEMIA

Two features set this disease apart from other leukemias: (1) inevitable and frequently severe hemorrhage from the time of inception and (2) the presence of numerous promyelocytes in the marrow.[1-3] The basis for the constant combination of these two features has been established—granules from disrupted promyelocytes release tissue thromboplastin, which promotes the consumption of serum clotting factors and platelets, the result being disseminated intravascular coagulation.

In the peripheral blood, pancytopenia is more common than leukocytosis. The decrease of developing red cells in the marrow, abetted by bleeding, is the basis for anemia, while the scarcity of megakaryocytes combined with accelerated intravascular consumption results in thrombocytopenia. In contrast to other acute leukemias, escape of immature white cells into the peripheral blood is limited, and leukopenia prevails in over 70 per cent of cases.

A distinctive chromosomal abnormality has been recognized in this disease, namely a translocation between chromosomes 15 and 17 t($15 q^+$; $17 q^-$).[4] In the United States the defect occurs in about one third of the cases. The presence of the defect conveys a poor prognosis. This is in contrast to the association of the Philadelphia chromosomal abnormality occurring in chronic granulocytic leukemia.

The diagnosis can be established with equal assurance from the core biopsy specimen and the smear of aspirated marrow particles (Fig. 2–5).[5] The marrow is completely or predominantly filled with promyelocytes. The prevailing standard for the diagnosis is that 50 per cent or more of the cells in the marrow be promyelocytes. A few myeloblasts, myelo-

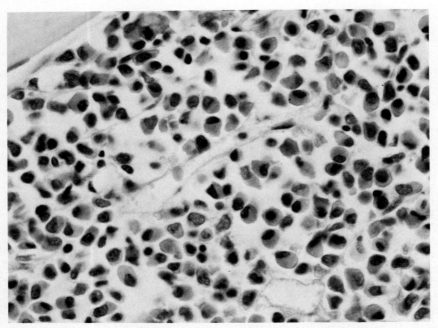

Figure 2–5. Malignant promyelocytes fill the marrow. With their eccentric nuclei and abundant cytoplasm, they may simulate abnormal plasma cells. 680×, H&E.

cytes, and neutrophils may be present, as may scattered megakaryocytes and groups of nucleated red cells. The promyelocyte is readily recognized in the core specimen section by abundant rust-colored cytoplasm surrounding the central or eccentric nucleus with its densely packed chromatin. The characteristic granules, *Auer bodies*, and spindly rods filling the cytoplasm, which are detectable in Wright-stained smear preparations, cannot be recognized in the sections. Despite this limitation, distinction of promyelocytic

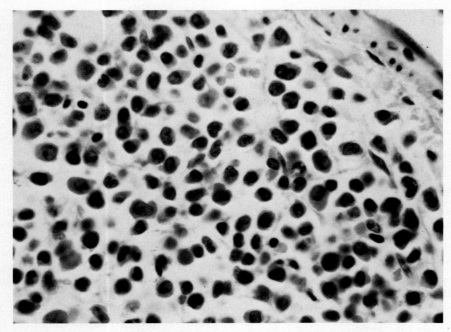

Figure 2–6. Microgranular variant of acute promyelocytic leukemia in which folding or lobation of the nuclei occurs. 680×, H&E.

leukemia from the other leukemias by the core specimen is rarely problematic. Differentiation from abnormal plasma cells in occasional cases of myeloma can be resolved by application of the immunoperoxidase technique.

A microgranular variant of acute promyelocytic leukemia has been described recently.[6, 7] The chief differences from the standard type are the marked leukocytosis rather than leukopenia in the peripheral blood, the ultrastructural dimensions of the cytoplasmic granules, and the folded or lobulated nucleus (Fig. 2–6). Hemorrhage is just as characteristic of the variant form as it is of the standard disease.

REFERENCES

1. Bennett, J. M., Catovsky, D., Daniel, M. T., et al.: Proposals for the classification of the acute leukemias. Br J Haematol 33:451–458, 1976.
2. Gralnick, H. R., and Tan, H. R.: Acute promyelocytic leukemia: A model for understanding the role of the malignant cell in hemostasis. Hum Pathol 5:661–673, 1974.
3. Groopman, J., and Ellman, L.: Acute promyelocytic leukemia. Am J Hematol 7:395–408, 1979.
4. Rowley, J. D., Golomb, H. M., and Dougherty, C.: 15/17 translocation. A consistent chromosomal change in acute promyelocytic leukaemia. Lancet 1:549–550, 1977.
5. Bernard, J., Lasneret, J., Chome, J., et al.: A cytological and histological study of acute premyelocytic leukemia. J Clin Pathol 16:319–324, 1963.
6. Bennett, J. M., Catovsky, D., Daniel, M. T., et al.: A variant form of hypergranular promyelocytic leukaemia (M3). Br J Haematol 44:169–170, 1980.
7. Savage, R. A., Hoffman, G. C., and Lucas, F. V.: Morphology and cytochemistry of "microgranular" acute promyelocytic leukemia (FAB M3m). Am J Clin Pathol 75:548–552, 1981.

ERYTHROLEUKEMIA (ACUTE ERYTHROBLASTIC LEUKEMIA)

The term "erythroleukemia" as used here is equated to the eponym *di Guglielmo syndrome*, a designation commonly used to include erythremic myelosis and erythroleukemia. In practice the distinction between erythremic myelosis and erythroleukemia is often imprecise, as is implicit in the use of the eponym, and thus is of doubtful therapeutic value. The term "erythroleukemia" clearly indicates the predominant cell lineage involved in this disease in a manner analogous to the nomenclature generally employed for the leukemias. In the French-American-British classification of acute leukemias the disease is designated as M-6.[1]

The disease is one of the least frequent of the leukemias in the myeloproliferative group.[2-4] It occurs de novo, occasionally in the wake of chronic granulocytic leukemia,[5] and rarely following polycythemia vera.[6]

The diagnosis can be established best from the characteristics of the marrow. Physical findings and abnormalities of the peripheral blood lack both consistency and specificity. For example, no more than half of the cases exhibit splenomegaly, and only about three fourths have pancytopenia with substantial numbers of circulating nucleated red blood cells and a few myeloblasts.

In evaluating the marrow in this disease the core biopsy specimen is secondary to the smear preparation in terms of informational content because of the dependence on subcellular detail for accurate assessment. In the core specimen nucleated red cells are overly abundant and are usually the dominant cell type (Figs. 2–7A, B, and C and 2–8). Maturation is abnormal in that the number of erythroblasts is increased, and early and intermediate normoblasts (basophilic and polychromatophilic) are more numerous than or as numerous as late normoblasts (orthochromatic). The erythroblast is recognized by its large size, a large vesicular nucleus containing nucleoli, and basophilic cytoplasm. When problematic, the distinction of the erythroblast and early normoblast from the myeloblast, monoblast, and plasmablast can tbe resolved by use of the immunoperoxidase method (Fig. 2–9).[7] The frequency of mitosis is above normal. Nuclear abnormalities in the form of multinucleation, lobation, and fragmentation may be discernible. Other stigmas, including megaloblastoid maturation, polyploidy, cytoplasmic vacuolation, and erythroblastic erythrophagocytosis, are better assessed in smear preparations. Cytoplasm glycogen accumulation as demonstrated by periodic acid-Schiff (PAS) positivity is common but not specific. It also occurs in megaloblastosis of vitamin B_{12} and folate deficiency and in intense normoblastic erythroid hyperplasia.

The number of granulocytes is decreased, especially the maturational forms beyond the myelocyte. Usually there is an increase in the number of myeloblasts, but this is overshadowed by the more numerous erythroblasts. The number of megakaryocytes is variable. Some may be qualitatively abnormal.

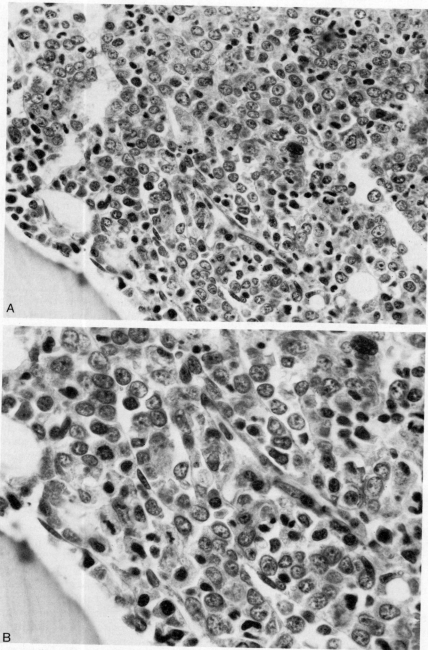

Figure 2–7. *A, B,* and *C.* The overwhelming majority of cells in this case of acute leukemia are erythroblasts. This cell approximates the size of a myeloblast and has a large round vesicular nucleus with dispersed granular chromatin. A small nucleolus is commonly evident. A ring of cytoplasm and distinct cell borders are also characteristic. In some cases assured distinction from the myeloblast or even the large transformed lymphocyte may require examination of a marrow smear preparation and use of cytochemical and immunocytochemical procedures. 400×, 680×, and 1000×, H&E.

Illustration continued on opposite page

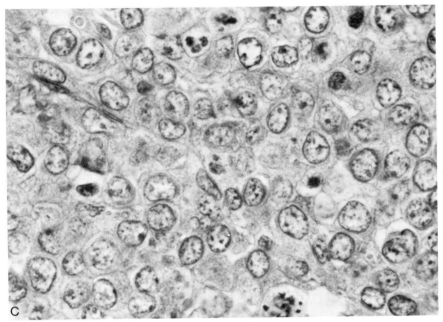

Figure 2–7. *Continued.*

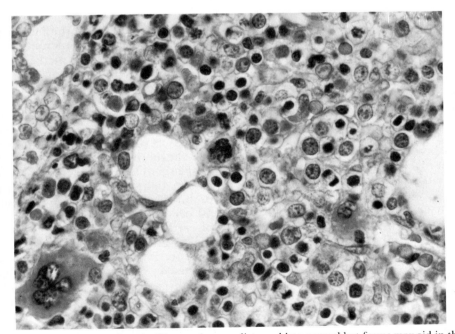

Figure 2–8. Foci of maturation of erythroblasts to intermediate and late normoblast forms may aid in the diagnosis of erythroleukemia, but if this is prevalent the picture may mimic pronounced megaloblastic erythroid hyperplasia. In this focus there are about equal numbers of early, intermediate, and late normoblasts and very few erythroblasts. The megakaryocytes are slightly atypical. 680×, H&E.

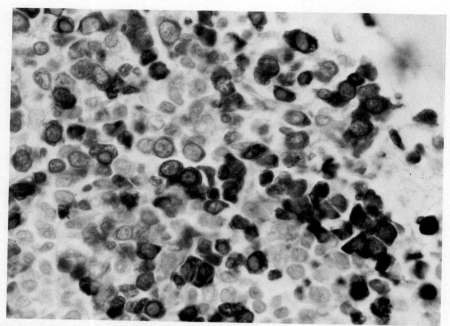

Figure 2–9. Demonstration of hemoglobin by the immunoperoxidase technique used for the definitive identification of erythroblasts in this case of acute leukemia. 680×, peroxidase antiperoxidase procedure.

Progression of the disease in most cases is manifested by an increasing number of myeloblasts relative to erythroblasts. Eventually the marrow is flooded with myeloblasts, and the condition is indistinguishable from acute myeloblastic leukemia. Rarely, only erythroblasts remain.

The differential diagnostic considerations include (1) other forms of acute leukemia, especially in the myeloid group, (2) treated leukemia, (3) idiopathic or drug-related myelodysplasia, and (4) megaloblastosis responsive to vitamins B_{12}, folate, or pyridoxine. The distinction of erythroleukemia from the other acute myeloid leukemias—namely myeloblastic, myelomonocytic, and monocytic leukemias—is difficult only when the latter have a disproportionate increase in erythroid proliferation with impaired maturation. When the erythroid increase is inordinate, the distinction of erythroleukemia from the other acute leukemias may rest on definitions. Erythroid abnormalities that on occasion become pronounced in the course of chemotherapy of nonerythroleukemias almost invariably recede on remission of the leukemia.

The distinction between erythroleukemia and myelodysplasia can be difficult, problematic, and at times arbitrary even when smear preparations of blood and marrow are evaluated in conjunction with the core biopsy specimen. Generally, the marrow section in myelodysplasia presents a far more variegated picture than that in erythroleukemia. Characteristically in myelodysplasia there is an obvious increase in the number of megakaryocytes, commonly micromegakaryocytes, in conjunction with the increase in erythroid cells, and maturational impairment in either erythroid or granulocytic lineages, or both, is invariable. As in the case of the differentiation of erythroleukemia from other acute leukemias, the distinction from myelodysplasia may revolve around definitions. The thesis that there can be a progression of myelodysplasia to leukemia depends on acceptance of the definitions of these diseases. When erythroblasts gain the ascendancy and exceed 50 per cent of the population, the diagnosis of erythroleukemia is virtually assured.

The distinction of erythroleukemia from B_{12}- and folate-dependent megaloblastosis is discussed in the section on anemia. Giant metamyelocytes or hypersegmented enlarged neutrophils are not present in the leukemia unless it is complicated by vitamin B_{12} or folate deficiency.

REFERENCES

1. Bennett, J. M., Catovsky, D., Daniel, M. T., et al.: Proposals for the classification of the acute leukemias. Br J Haematol 33:451–458, 1976.

2. Henderson, E. S.: Acute myelogenous leukemia. *In* Williams, W. J., Beutler, E., Erslev, A. J., and Lichtman, M. A. (eds.): Hematology. New York, McGraw-Hill, 1983, pp. 239–253.
3. Sondergaard-Petersen, H.: The diGuglielmo syndrome. Acta Med Scand 198:165–174, 1975.
4. Roggli, V. L., and Saleem, A.: Erythroleukemia. Cancer 49:101–108, 1982.
5. Rosenthal, S., Canellos, G. P., and Gralnick, H. R.: Erythroblastic transformation of chronic granulocytic leukemia. Am J Med 63:116–124, 1977.
6. Bank, A., Larsen, P. R., and Anderson, H. M.: diGuglielmo's syndrome after polycythemia. N Engl J Med 275:489–490, 1966.
7. Pinkus, G. S., and Said, J. W.: Intracellular hemoglobin—a specific marker for erythroid cells in paraffin sections. Am J Pathol 102:308–313, 1981.

ACUTE MEGAKARYOCYTIC LEUKEMIA

This leukemia is among the least common of the leukemias, and an occurrence of this disease continues to merit the status of a "reportable case." Only since the innovation of a procedure for the specific ultrastructural cytochemical identification of the megakaryoblast has the precursor of the megakaryocyte been clearly distinguishable from its allied blast cell counterparts.[1] Prior to this development, the only reliable evidence for acute megakaryocytic leukemia was the demonstration of myriads of mature but bizarre and grotesque megakaryocytes and of micromegakaryocytes in the marrow. Acceptable cases based on this morphology are exemplified by those reported by Rappaport[2] and Kajita.[3] By contrast, current methodology, which includes immunomorphological[4-6] and ultrastructural cytochemical[1] procedures has facilitated the detection of megakaryoblasts and thereby made possible the diagnosis of megakaryoblast crisis in chronic granulocytic leukemia[7] and in chronic primary myelofibrosis[1] as well as of acute megakaryocytic leukemia de novo.[5] These advances have led to the suggestion that acute megakaryocytic leukemia be added to the French-American-British classification of acute leukemias and be designated as M-7.[8]

Most of the authentic cases of acute megakaryocytic leukemia have occurred in adults over the age of 50 years, but infants and young adults have also been afflicted. Absence of organ enlargement initially is the rule, as is generally true in acute leukemia. Typically there is pancytopenia with profound thrombocytopenia. Varying numbers of blast cells, usually less than 25 per cent of the circulating white cells, are in the blood and by the aforementioned techniques have been shown to be megakaryoblasts. Few, if any, micromegakaryocytes or megakaryocytes circulate, despite their abundance in the marrow. This disparity has been emphasized as a characteristic of the disease.[5]

Typically little or no marrow can be aspirated. This fact can be attributed to the presence of a dense reticulin mesh enveloping the marrow cells. Therefore, the marrow core biopsy may be essential to establish the diagnosis. The preponderant cell lineage is megakaryocytic, with varying admixtures of megakaryoblasts, micromegakaryocytes, and more or less dysplastic megakaryocytes (Figs. 2–10*A*, *B*, and *C*). Developing granulocytes and red cells are decreased in number and generally overwhelmed by the dominating megakaryocytic lineage. Although reticulin is abundant, there is no collagen fibrosis.

Problems in the differential diagnosis of acute megakaryoblastic leukemia are related to confusion with (1) acute myeloblastic leukemia or erythroleukemia with somewhat increased numbers of atypical megakaryocytes or of micromegakaryocytes, (2) megakaryoblastic crisis in chronic granulocytic leukemia, in chronic primary myelofibrosis, and possibly in essential thrombocythemia, (3) acute myelodysplasia, and (4) malignant myelosclerosis. For diseases in the first and second groups characterization of the dominant blast population by cytochemical or immunocytochemical methods can resolve enigmatic cases. The third and fourth groups are more difficult to differentiate because diverse definitions compound the complexity of morphological features. Recent publications have proposed that malignant myelosclerosis is identical to acute megakaryocytic leukemia.[9, 10] Other authors have denied this claim, maintaining that malignant myelosclerosis is a disease sui generis.[11] A recent analytical review of malignant myelosclerosis emphasized the factitious inclusion of leukemias complicated by collagen fibrosis in this disease category, especially acute myeloblastic leukemia.[12] This analysis, however, has in turn been criticized by the assertion that acute myelodysplasia was misidentified as malignant myelosclerosis.[11] The assertion averred that the original description of malignant myelosclerosis describes the marrow morphology as identical to chronic myelofibrosis[13] and that this criterion was not used in the analytical review. Although additional study of cases is necessary, the facts that reticulin and collagen fibrosis in the marrow

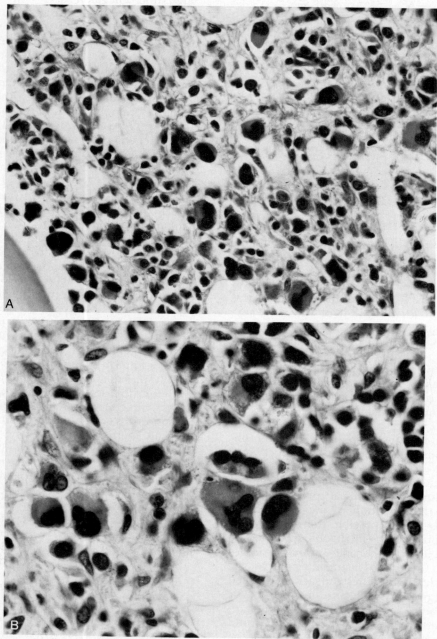

Figure 2–10. *A, B,* and *C.* Numerous abnormal megakaryocytes are scattered through a delicate fibrillary stromal background in the company of smaller blast cells and immature forms of the granulocytic and erythroid lines. The megakaryocytes have larger, nonlobated but sometimes more complex nuclei than the micromegakaryocytes. They are not, however, as bizarre or as pleomorphic as those in chronic primary myelofibrosis. 400×, 680×, and 680×, H&E.

Illustration continued on opposite page

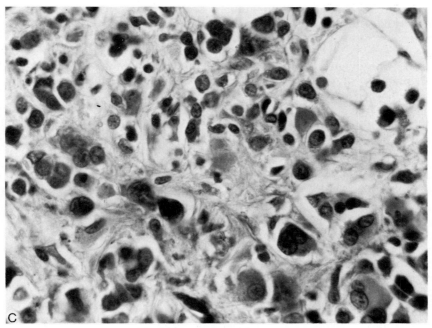

Figure 2–10. *Continued.*

are reactive and nonspecific rather than neoplastic[14] and that megakaryocytes can induce fibroplasia in any setting[15] support the view that malignant myelosclerosis is not a disease entity and that reported cases so designated represent various diseases, including acute megakaryocytic leukemia, acute myelodysplasia, and possibly acute myeloblastic leukemia or erythroleukemia with a high content of atypical megakaryocytes or micromegakaryocytes and collagen fibrosis.

REFERENCES

1. Breton-Gorius, J., Daniel, M. T., Flandrin, G., et al.: Fine structure of peroxidase activity of circulating micromegakaryocytes and platelets in a case of acute myelofibrosis. Br J Haematol 25:331–339, 1973.
2. Rappaport, H.: Tumors of the hematopoietic system. *In* Atlas of Tumor Pathology. Section 3. Fascicle 8. Washington, D.C., Armed Forces Institute of Pathology, 1966, pp. 294–300.
3. Kajita, A., and Hirokawa, K.: An autopsy case of a leukemic megakaryocytosis. Acta Pathol Jpn 23:421–430, 1973.
4. Ching-Hon, P., Williams, D. L., Scarborough, V., et al.: Acute megakaryocytic leukemia associated with intrinsic platelet dysfunction and constitutional ring 21 chromosome in a young boy. Br. J Haematol 50:191–200, 1982.
5. Bevan, D., Rose, M., and Greaves, M.: Leukaemia of platelet precursors: Diverse features in four cases. Br J Haematol 51:147–164, 1982.
6. Innes, D. J., Mills, S. E., and Walker, G. K.: Mega-karyocytic leukemia. Am J Clin Pathol 77:107–110, 1982.
7. Bain, B., Catovsky, D., O'Brien, M., et al.: Megakaryoblastic transformation of chronic granulocytic leukemia. J Clin Pathol 30:235–242, 1977.
8. Kay, H. E. M.: Acute leukemia. *In* Hoffbrand, A. V. (ed.): Recent Advances in Haematology. Edinburgh, Churchill Livingstone, 1982, p. 165.
9. den Ottolander, G. J., te Velde, J., Brederoo, P., et al.: Megakaryoblastic leukaemia (acute myelofibrosis): A report of three cases. Br J Haematol 42:9–20, 1979.
10. Bain, B. J., Catovsky, D., O'Brien, M., et al.: Megakaryoblastic leukemia presenting as acute myelofibrosis—a study of four cases with the platelet-peroxidase reaction. Blood 58:206–213, 1981.
11. Sultan, C., Sigaux, F., Imbert, M., et al.: Acute myelodysplasia with myelofibrosis: A report of eight cases. Br J Haematol 49:11–16, 1981.
12. Bearman, R. M., Pangalis, G. A., and Rappaport, H.: Acute (malignant) myelosclerosis. Cancer 43:279–293, 1979.
13. Lewis, S. M., and Szur, L.: Malignant myelosclerosis. Br Med J 2:472–477, 1963.
14. Jacobson, R. J., Salo, A., and Fialkow, P. J.: Agnogenic myeloid metaplasia: A clonal proliferation of hematopoietic stem cells with secondary myelofibrosis. Blood 51:189–194, 1978.
15. Castro-Malaspina, H., Rabellino, E. M., Yen, A., et al.: Human megakaryocytic stimulation of proliferation of bone marrow fibroblasts. Blood 57:781–787, 1981.

CHRONIC GRANULOCYTIC LEUKEMIA

Most cases of chronic granulocytic leukemia are readily recognized. In an adult when splenomegaly is combined with mild anemia and marked granulocytosis in which a melange of developing and mature neutrophils is accompanied by basophilia in the peripheral blood, the diagnosis is almost assured.[1-3] The majority of problematic cases arise when the spleen is not enlarged or the granulocytosis does not exceed 50,000 cells per microliter. Finding the neutrophilic alkaline phosphatase activity depressed and the Philadelphia chromosomal defect present resolves the diagnosis of most equivocal cases.

The marrow core biopsy is usually an adjunctive rather than a requisite procedure in the diagnosis. The cellularity of the marrow is markedly increased. As a rule, the entire intertrabecular space is packed with hematopoietic cells. Typically myelocytes occupy the peritrabecular zone, and neutrophils and band forms fill the midzone (Fig. 2–11). Myelocytes also surround small arteries and veins and less commonly the sinusoids. The immature granulocyte cells characteristically adhere to one another, whereas neutrophils tend to dissociate into individual cells. This lack of cohesion of neutrophils in conjunction with little, if any, increase in reticulin fibers commonly results in a fragmented core specimen. In some cases the number of eosinophilic myelocytes is conspicuously increased. Basophils, characteristically increased in number, are not visualized when the tissue is fixed in aqueous solution. By definition, myeloblasts do not exceed 5 per cent of the granulocyte population. The number of normoblasts is decidedly decreased, either absolutely or relatively, and they are present in small infrequent clusters. Erythroid maturation is normal. Megakaryocytes are present in variable numbers, ranging from markedly decreased in many cases, to essentially normal in some, slightly increased in a few (Fig. 2–12), and greatly increased in an exceptional instance. Qualitative alteration of the megakaryocytes is common but rarely of the magnitude so characteristic of chronic primary myelofibrosis or even of polycythemia vera or essential thrombocythemia. Thus, in chronic granulocyte leukemia among the normal and randomly distributed megakaryocytes there is an occasional cell with little or no cytoplasm, an occasional coherent diad or triad of mature megakaryocytes, or a few with nonlobated nuclei. The latter situation may be more apparent than real because additional nuclear lobes may be present beyond the plane of the tissue section. In the exceptional case, perhaps one or two in a hundred, there is a high content of immature megakaryocytes or micromegakaryocytes (Fig. 2–13). These cases may represent codominance of granu-

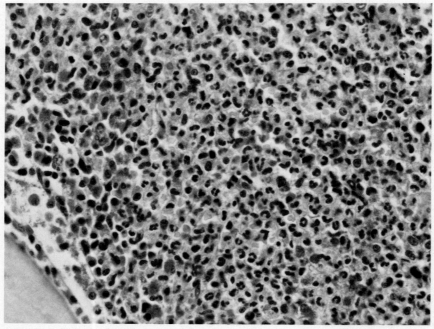

Figure 2–11. The intertrabecular space is filled with granulocytes to the virtual exclusion of other hematopoietic cells. The majority are mature. Myelocytes are most obvious adjacent to the bone trabecula. 400×, H&E.

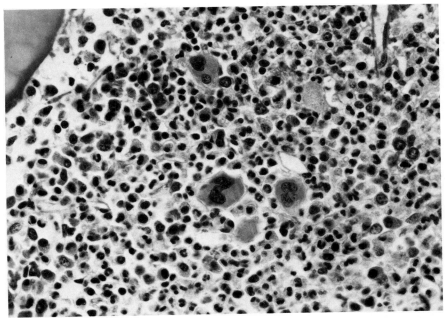

Figure 2–12. A slightly increased number of megakaryocytes, which are at most slightly altered morphologically, are present among the numerous granulocytes. 400×, H&E.

locyte and megakaryocyte lineages in the initial stages of the disease or, as noted later, a megakaryocytic type of progression occurring at a relatively early stage. A few macrophages closely simulating Gaucher's cells are present in about 20 per cent of cases (Figs. 2–14 and 2–15).[4] Macrophages also may contain other debris, but hemosiderin is usually not present. Bone trabeculae, as a rule, are normal.

The inevitable evolution of the disease from the chronic to the blast phase occurs

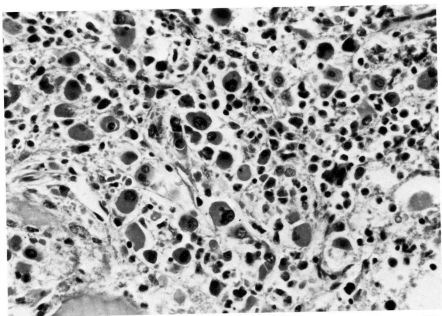

Figure 2–13. A large number of micromegakaryocytes are among the granulocytes in the case of Ph′ (+) chronic granulocytic leukemia. Micromegakaryocytes have nonlobated or bilobated nuclei and a moderate amount of cytoplasm. 400×, H&E.

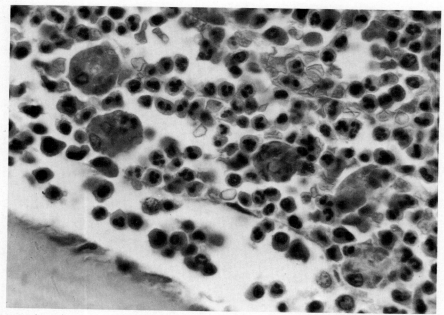

Figure 2–14. Formative stage of pseudo-Gaucher's cells in chronic granulocytic leukemia. Ingested neutrophils are evident in some histiocytes, while other histiocytes have advanced to the wrinkled cytoplasm stage. 680×, H&E.

abruptly or gradually through an accelerated stage.[1,3,5] The core specimen is useful in evaluating these phase changes and in particular the efficacy of more intensive chemotherapy. Progression of the disease is manifested in the marrow by a shift from the preponderance of neutrophils and band forms to an increasing proportion of myelocytes and blast cells and finally to a population predominately of blast cells. When the latter stage is reached there is no morphological distinction from acute leukemia beginning as such. The exception to this is the presence of pseudo-Gaucher's cells in mar-

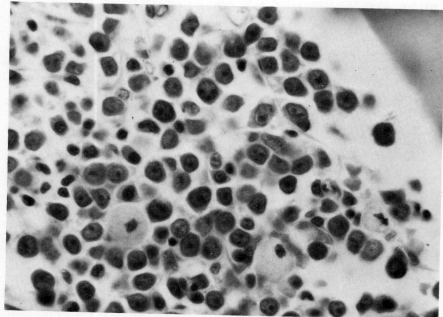

Figure 2–15. Myeloblasts fill the marrow in the blast crisis of Ph′ (+) chronic granulocytic leukemia whose prior existence is betrayed by the pseudo-Gaucher's cells. 680×, H&E.

row that contains an excessive number of myeloblasts (Fig. 2–15). This has been found only in cases preceded by chronic granulocytic leukemia. In most cases the blast cells are myeloid, but in some they are distinctly lymphoid.[2, 5] The latter are usually B-lymphoblasts.[6] In unusual cases there is evolution to the megakaryocytic[7–9] and rarely to the normoblastic lineage.[10]

A mild increase in stromal reticulin fibers is common in the chronic phase. This increase is nonspecific and occurs to varying degrees in many forms of leukemia and lymphoma.[11, 12] Pronounced degrees have been designated "reticulin fibrosis" and may be the basis of nonproductive aspiration of the marrow.[13] This condition is exceptional in the chronic phase. Marked reticulin fibrosis and focal and mild collagen fibrosis may be found in the accelerated and blast phases (Fig. 2–16).[14] This is unrelated to any associated increase in recognizable megakaryocytes except in the unusual case of megakaryocytic evolution (Fig. 2–17). However, pronounced collagen fibrosis commonly develops during intensive chemotherapy of the blast crisis.[15–17] After remission has been achieved the collagen fibrosis may not be demonstrable in subsequent core specimens. This fibrosis is distinctly different from that of chronic primary myelofibrosis by virtue of the entrapped bizarre megakaryocytes in the latter disease.

This fibrosis also differs from that of Philadelphia-chromosome–positive chronic granulocytic leukemia in megakaryocytic evolution, in which immature megakaryocytes or micromegakaryocytes prevail. Failure to recognize these differences has served to foster the unsubstantiated notion that chronic granulocytic leukemia converts to chronic primary myelofibrosis.

Differential diagnostic considerations include some of the diseases in the myeloproliferative group and reactive granulocytosis. In polycythemia vera normoblasts are usually more abundant and at least as numerous as granulocytes. Megakaryocytes are usually more numerous in polycythemia vera. Essential thrombocythemia is distinguished by the mass of megakaryocytes present. The distinction from chronic primary myelofibrosis has been alluded to already. In chronic myelomonocytic leukemia the cell population is more heterogeneous, and myelocytes and monocytes are far more numerous than mature neutrophils. Most problems in interpreting the core specimen in this disease arise with or follow therapy of the accelerated or blast phase.

In reactive granulocytosis the cellularity is rarely greater than 75 to 80 per cent (Fig. 2–18). This level always is exceeded in the untreated chronic phase of the disease, which is the only phase that requires consideration

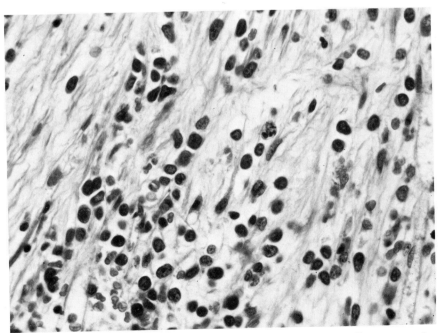

Figure 2–16. Blastic progression of chronic granulocytic leukemia in which blast cells permeate through a bed of collagen. 520×, H&E.

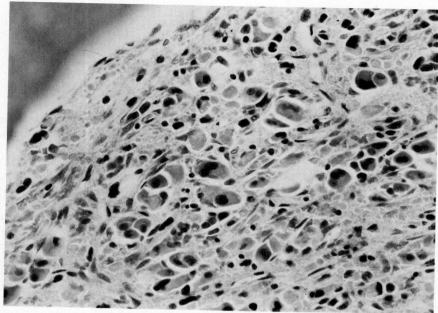

Figure 2–17. Large numbers of micromegakaryocytes are accompanied by and enclosed within collagen in megakaryocytic evolution of Ph′ (+) chronic granulocytic leukemia. Megakaryoblasts and myeloblasts cannot be distinguished clearly from each other in the standard section of the core specimen. 325×, H&E.

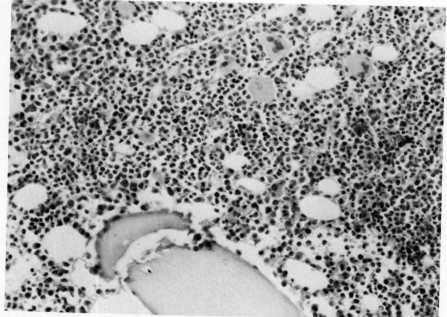

Figure 2–18. The persistence of fat cells in the marrow space is an important clue for distinguishing granulocytic hyperplasia from untreated chronic granulocytic leukemia in which virtually all fat cells are displaced. 250×, H&E.

in this context. An exception to this is the rare case of hypereosinophilic syndrome in which a markedly hypercellular marrow contains excessive numbers of eosinophilic myelocytes, metamyelocytes, and mature granulocytes. In this case the distinction from chronic eosinophilic leukemia may depend on the presence or absence of the Philadelphia or other types of chromosomal defect.[18]

REFERENCES

1. Rundles, R. W.: Chronic myelogenous leukemia. *In* Williams, W. J., Beutler, E., Erslev, A. J., and Lichtman, M. A. (eds.): Hematology. New York, McGraw-Hill, 1983, pp. 196–214.
2. Kamada, N., and Uchino, H.: Chronologic sequence in appearance of clinical and laboratory findings characteristic of chronic myelocytic leukemia. Blood 51:843–850, 1978.
3. Koeffler, H. P., and Golde, D. W.: Chronic myelogenous leukemia—new concepts. N Engl J Med 304:1201–1209, 1981.
4. Lee, R. E., and Ellis, L. D.: The storage cells of chronic myelogenous leukemia. Lab Invest 24:261–264, 1971.
5. Spiers, A. S. D.: Metamorphosis of chronic granulocytic leukemia: Diagnosis, classification, and management. Br J Haematol 41:1–7, 1979.
6. Bakhshi, A., Minowada, J., Arnold, A., et al.: Lymphoid blast crises of chronic myelogenous leukemia represent stages in the development of B-cell precursors. N Engl J Med 309:826–831, 1983.
7. Bain, B., Catovsky, D., O'Brien, M., et al.: Megakaryoblastic transformation of chronic granulocytic leukemia: An electron microscopy and cytochemical study. J Clin Pathol 30:235–242, 1977.
8. Breton-Gorius, J., Reyes, F., Vernant, J. P., et al.: The blast crisis of chronic granulocytic leukaemia: Megakaryoblastic nature of cells as revealed by the presence of platelet-peroxidase—a cytochemical ultrastructural study. Br J Haematol 39:295–303, 1978.
9. Williams, W. C., and Weiss, G. B.: Megakaryoblastic transformation of chronic myelogenous leukemia. Cancer 49:921–926, 1982.
10. Rosenthal, S., Canellos, G. P., and Gralnick, H. R.: Erythroblastic transformation of chronic granulocytic leukemia. Am J Med 63:116–124, 1977.
11. Burston, J., and Pinniger, J. L.: The reticulin content of bone marrow in haematological disorders. Br J Haematol 9:172–184, 1963.
12. Sanerkin, N. G.: Stromal changes in leukaemic and related bone marrow proliferation. J Clin Pathol 17:541–547, 1964.
13. Kundel, D. W., Brecher, G., Bodey, G. P., et al.: Reticulin fibrosis and bone infarction in acute leukemia. Implications for prognosis. Blood 23:526–544, 1964.
14. Gralnick, H. R., Harbor, J., and Vogel, C.: Myelofibrosis in chronic granulocytic leukemia. Blood 37:152–162, 1971.
15. Buyssens, N., and Bourgeois, N. H.: Chronic myelocytic leukemia versus idiopathic myelofibrosis. A diagnostic problem in bone marrow biopsies. Cancer 40:1548–1561, 1977.
16. Clough, V., Geary, C. G., Hashmi, K., et al.: Myelofibrosis in chronic granulocytic leukemia. Br J Haematol 42:515–526, 1979.
17. Wittels, B.: Bone marrow biopsy changes following chemotherapy for acute leukemia. Am J Surg Pathol 4:135–142, 1980.
18. Zucker-Franklin, D.: Eosinopenia and eosinophilia. *In* Williams, W. J., Beutler, E., Erslev, A. J., and Lichtman, M. A. (eds.): Hematology. New York, McGraw-Hill, 1983, pp. 825–828.

CHRONIC MYELOMONOCYTIC AND MONOCYTIC LEUKEMIAS

Paralleling the recognized types of acute leukemia that form the myeloid group are these two types of chronic leukemia, which are related to but usually distinctly different from chronic granulocytic leukemia.[1-3] Whereas the acute forms of these leukemias are relatively common, especially the myelomonocytic type, the chronic forms are uncommon, with the monocytic form being rare. Some cases have been misinterpreted as Philadelphia-chromosome–negative granulocytic leukemia. Although the FAB Cooperative Group classifies chronic myelomonocytic leukemia as a form of myelodysplasia, it continues to designate the disease as a leukemia.[4]

Monocytosis is typically present in the blood in both of these leukemias. The marrow is hypercellular and laden with monocytes, myelocytes, or both (Fig. 2–19). Smaller numbers of their precursor cells may be present. Associated abnormalities of erythroid and megakaryocytic maturation are common. Distinction of these leukemias, especially the myelomonocytic type, from myelodysplasia may be problematic and depend on definitions. Identification of myelocytes and monocytes in the marrow core specimen can be facilitated by cyto- and immunocytochemical procedures. The presence of lysozyme identifies the mononuclear cells as belonging to the monocyte-granulocyte lineage, and the Leder stain assists in distinguishing between the monocyte and the myelocyte divisions.

Aside from myelodysplasia and other forms of leukemia, the differential diagnostic considerations include selective neutropenia, either autoimmune or drug-related, and unusual instances of a reconstituting marrow after chemotherapy for acute leukemia. In selective neutropenia the marrow may be moderately hypercellular and display a striking preponderance of myelocytes with a lack of more mature granulocytes (Fig. 2–20). The other lineages, however, are unaffected

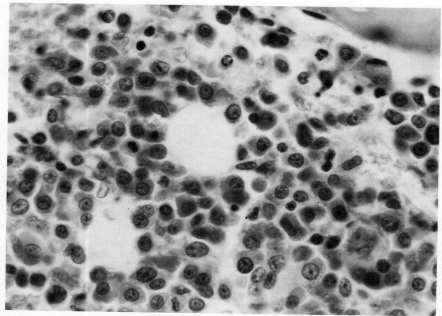

Figure 2–19. Chronic myelomonocytic leukemia was manifested by profound neutropenia in an elderly man whose hypercellular marrow has a superabundance of myelocytes but a dearth of more mature granulocytes. There was no organ enlargement. He subsequently developed anemia and thrombocytopenia, followed by acute leukemia. 680×, H&E.

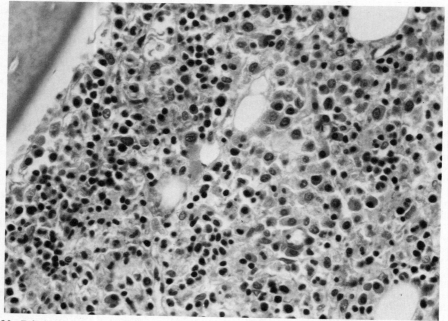

Figure 2–20. Felty's syndrome with an elevated granulocyte antibody titer was found in a man experiencing repeated infections. The highly cellular marrow has a normal myeloid-to-erythroid ratio with a normal maturation in the red cell series but a striking paucity of granulocyte members beyond the myelocyte level. 400×, H&E.

in contrast to the leukemias and myelodysplasias. In an occasional case of treated leukemia the granulocyte lineage in the repopulating marrow may predominate and not have matured beyond the myelocyte stage at the time of biopsy. Other features commonly present in the reconstituting marrow, the history of treated leukemia, and evidence of complete granulocyte maturation in a specimen obtained five to ten days later serve to clarify the diagnosis.

REFERENCES

1. Geary, C. G., Catovsky, D., Wiltshaw, E., et al.: Chronic myelomonocytic leukemia. Br J Haematol 30:289–302, 1975.
2. Zittoun, R.: Subacute and chronic myelomonocytic leukaemia: A distinct haematological entity. Br J Haematol 32:1–7, 1976.
3. Bearman, R. M., Kjeldsberg, C. R., Pangalis, G. A., et al.: Chronic monocytic leukemia in adults. Cancer 48:2239–2255, 1981.
4. Bennett, J. M., Catovsky, D., Daniel, M. T., et al.: Proposals for the classification of the myelodysplastic syndromes. Br J Haematol 51:189–199, 1982.

POLYCYTHEMIA VERA (CHRONIC ERYTHROCYTIC LEUKEMIA)

Stringent criteria have been formulated for the diagnosis of polycythemia vera.[1] An absolute increase in red cell mass with a normal arterial oxygen saturation is mandatory. Typically there is splenomegaly, but if the spleen is not enlarged, at least two of the following features must be present to satisfy the diagnostic requirements: thrombocytosis, leukocytosis with absolute neutrophilia, elevated leukocyte alkaline phosphatase score, and elevated serum B_{12} concentration or binding capacity. Utilizing these criteria for selection of cases, the Polycythemia Vera Study Group has delineated the features and variations present in the marrow core specimen before treatment.[2] For assessing the marrow in this disease the core specimen is superior to smears of aspirated marrow particles; in fact, the latter have been considered to be of little value.

Characteristically the marrow is hypercellular owing to an increase in the erythroid, granulocytic, and megakaryocytic lineages (Fig. 2–21). The mean cellularity in the series studied by the Polycythemia Vera Study Group was 82 per cent. Of note, however, is the observation that in 13 per cent of the cases the cellularity was assessed as normal or only slightly increased, that is, between 35 and 60 per cent. Thus, the lack of marrow hypercellularity does not exclude the diagnosis of polycythemia vera.

The myeloid-erythroid ratio in the marrow is typically altered because of a normoblastic erythroid proliferation. At least early in the course of the disease marrow erythroid pro-

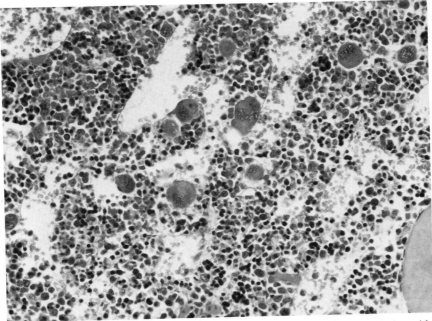

Figure 2–21. In the typical case the marrow is hypercellular and punctuated by dilated sinusoids. Normoblasts predominate, and megakaryocytes are moderately increased in number and somewhat atypical. 250×, H&E.

duction is effective, and the red cells produced have a normal life span.[1] Basophilic and polychromatophilic normoblasts are more numerous than in the normal state and in some cases may even prevail over orthochromatic forms (Fig. 2–22). This may be related to depletion of marrow iron stores, which is characteristic of the disease and which was present in over 90 per cent of cases in the Polycythemia Vera Study Group series. Therefore, the presence or absence of hemosiderin in the marrow can be of diagnostic significance.

In the same series the number of megakaryocytes was moderately to markedly increased in approximately 75 per cent of cases. But some 25 per cent of cases showed a normal or only slightly increased number of megakaryocytes (Fig. 2–23). Whether increased in number or not, megakaryocytes usually occur as singlets rather than as coherent clusters and exhibit only minimal or at most moderate deviation from normal morphology (Figs. 2–21 and 2–23). Increased amounts of cytoplasm and some nuclear atypia or complexity are the rule, but bizarre forms as occur in chronic primary myelofibrosis are uncommon. Two studies have indicated an average increase in megakaryocyte volume of approximately 40 per cent.[3, 4] This translates into an increase in cross-sectional area of about 20 per cent and an average

increase in diameter of about 10 per cent. Nuclear lobes are proportionately increased. Occasionally a megakaryocyte in mitosis is present. Despite their neoplastic character, the megakaryocytes efficiently and effectively produce platelets with a normal life span.[3]

Granulocytes and precursors are almost always less numerous than normoblasts. Their maturation is normal.

The reticulin fiber content of the marrow has been studied repeatedly in the normal and abnormal marrow.[5–8] The quality or quantity of these fibers is never diagnostic of any disease, nor do any deviations from the normal necessarily lend support or confirmation to a particular diagnosis. In 88 per cent of untreated cases in the Polycythemia Vera Study Group series reticulin was judged to be normal or slightly increased. While the amount of reticulin may increase in a given case, this change does not necessarily indicate a progression from the stable to the spent phase of the disease. Increases in reticulin, when they do occur, are almost certainly a reactive response and not a neoplastic fibroplasia.[9, 10]

In about half the cases the marrow sinusoids are conspicuously dilated and contain normoblasts or megakaryocytes, or both (Figs. 2–21 and 2–24).

The effect of treatment on marrow morphology is difficult to assess because post-

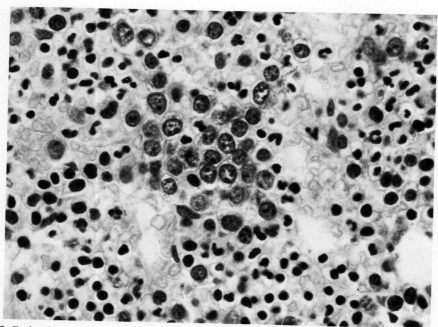

Figure 2–22. Early- (large cells) and intermediate-stage normoblasts may be as abundant as late-stage (small cells) normoblasts. 680×, H&E.

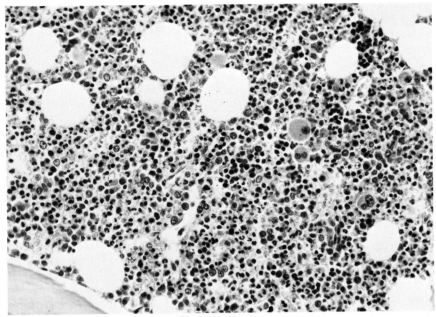

Figure 2–23. In some cases cellularity is less than 100 per cent, as indicated by persistence of fat cells, and the number of megakaryocytes is not increased. The morphological distinction from erythrocytosis and compensatory erythroid hyperplasia is not possible in these cases. 250×, H&E.

therapeutic biopsy is usually done only after unusual features appear in the blood. Phlebotomy appears to have little effect on cellularity, while phosphorus-32 (^{32}P) and melphalan decrease it. The drugs also appear to induce bizarre megakaryocyte morphology akin to that more commonly present in chronic primary myelofibrosis.

Polycythemia vera can be complicated by marrow fibrosis or can progress to acute myeloblastic leukemia.[1, 11, 12] On occasion both conditions develop in the same patient. The

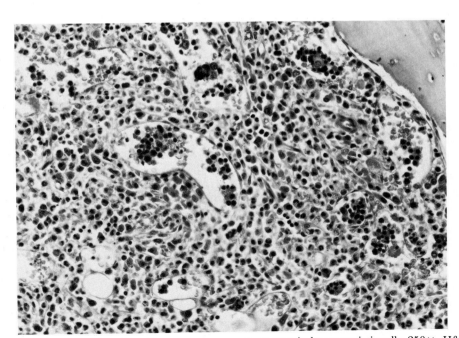

Figure 2–24. The gaping sinusoids may appear empty or contain hematopoietic cells. 250×, H&E.

diagnosis of postpolycythemic myelofibrosis is tenable only when collagen with entrapment of megakaryocytes is demonstrable in the core biopsy specimen. This occurs in as many as 25 per cent of cases after an average of ten years of polycythemia vera.[11] Acute leukemia develops in as many as 14 per cent of cases.[11] A recent report documents the observation that therapy influences the rate of its occurrence; significantly higher rates of leukemia occur with chlorambucil than with phlebotomy or ^{32}P treatment.[12]

Differential considerations in the diagnosis of polycythemia vera include stress erythrocytosis; erythrocytosis of inappropriate erythropoietin production as occurs in certain tumors and renal lesions; compensatory erythroid hyperplasia of hemolysis, blood loss, and hypoxia; essential thrombocythemia; and chronic granulocytic leukemia. In erythrocytosis and erythroid hyperplasia orthochromatic normoblasts dominate the hypercellular marrow, and megakaryocytes are normal or only slightly increased in number; in thrombocythemia masses of megakaryocytes are the striking feature; in chronic granulocytic leukemia granulocytic proliferation is predominant, although the number of megakaryocytes may be increased. These differences are distinctive in most cases. In some cases, however, they are not, and the diagnosis of polycythemia vera cannot be based solely on, or clearly excluded by, the features present in the marrow.

REFERENCES

1. Murphy, S.: Polycythemia vera. *In* Williams, W. J., Beutler, E., Erslev, A. J., and Lichtman, M. A. (eds.): Hematology. New York, McGraw-Hill, 1983, pp. 185–196.
2. Ellis, J. T., and Peterson, P.: The bone marrow in polycythemia vera. *In* Sommers, S. C. (ed.): Pathology Annual. Vol. 14. Part 1. New York, Appleton-Century-Crofts, 1979, pp. 383–403.
3. Harker, L. A., and Finch, C. A.: Thrombokinetics in man. J Clin Invest 48:963–974, 1969.
4. Kutti, J., Ridell, B., Weinfeld, A., et al.: The relation of thrombokinetics to bone marrow megakaryocytes and to the size of the spleen in polycythaemia vera. Scand J Haematol 10:88–95, 1973.
5. Burston, J., and Pinniger, J. L.: The reticulin content of bone marrow in haematological disorders. Br J Haematol 9:172–184, 1963.
6. Sanerkin, N. G.: Stromal changes in leukaemic and related bone marrow proliferation. J Clin Pathol 17:541–547, 1964.
7. Roberts, B. E., Miles, D. W., and Woods, C. G.: Polycythaemia vera and myelosclerosis: A bone marrow study. Br J Haematol 16:75–85, 1969.
8. Lennert, K., Nagai, K., and Schwarze, E. W.: Pathological features of the bone marrow. *In* Videback, A. (ed.): Clin Haematol 4:331–351, 1975.
9. Adamson, J. W., and Fialkow, P. J.: The pathogenesis of myeloproliferative syndromes. Br J Haematol 38:299–303, 1978.
10. Groopman, J. E.: The pathogenesis of myelofibrosis in myeloproliferative disorders. Ann Intern Med 92:857–858, 1980.
11. Gunz, F., and Baikie, A. G.: Leukemia. 3rd ed. New York, Grune & Stratton, 1974, pp. 377–430.
12. Berk, P. D., Goldberg, J. D., Silverstein, M. N., et al.: Increased incidence of acute leukemia in polycythemia vera associated with chlorambucil therapy. N Engl J Med 304:441–447, 1981.

ESSENTIAL THROMBOCYTHEMIA (CHRONIC MEGAKARYOCYTIC LEUKEMIA)

The most remarkable and characteristic features of this uncommon disease are a prodigious and persistent elevation of platelets in the blood to levels in excess of one million per microliter and a profusion of megakaryocytes in the marrow.[1] As could be expected, this degree of thrombocytosis is manifested clinically by recurrent episodes of hemorrhage and thrombosis. The bleeding is usually from the gastrointestinal or urogenital tract. Rarely is there purpura. The thrombosis most commonly involves the splenic vein or the leg veins. The splenic vein thrombosis with its consequent infarction and atrophy of the spleen can account for the absence of splenomegaly, which is otherwise present in many cases. Signs of cerebral or basilar-vertebral artery thrombosis are also frequent.

In addition to the pronounced thrombocytosis in the blood, there is usually a mild neutrophilia. In the event of chronic bleeding, hypochromic anemia is present; in the absence of bleeding or iron deficiency, there may be mild erythrocytosis. The presence of various red cell inclusions signifies splenic hypofunction following splenic atrophy.[2]

The marrow core specimen is most useful in reliably evaluating the cellularity and the megakaryocyte population in this disease (Figs. 2–25 and 2–26). The cellularity varies greatly, ranging from 100 per cent to as low as 25 per cent. The most consistent and dependable diagnostic feature is the overwhelming number of megakaryocytes placed in a background of normally maturing granulocytes. Even when the cellularity is low, the overabundance of megakaryocytes is obvious. Clustering of the megakaryocytes and mild to moderate degrees of cytological atypia are

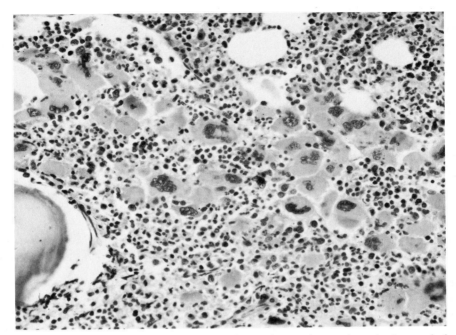

Figure 2–25. Numerous megakaryocytes are closely clustered or coherent in a background dominated by granulocytes. Most are enlarged and possess a complex lobated nucleus, and a few are small and have simplified nonlobated or bilobated nuclei. 250×, H&E.

common features, whereas marked dysplasia or denudation of nuclei is unusual. Many of the megakaryocytes are enlarged by increases in cytoplasm and nuclear lobations. Megakaryocytes in mitosis may be present. Despite their neoplastic character, the megakaryocytes maintain effective platelet production.[3]

Small foci of collagen fibrosis are rarely present. Such foci may signal development

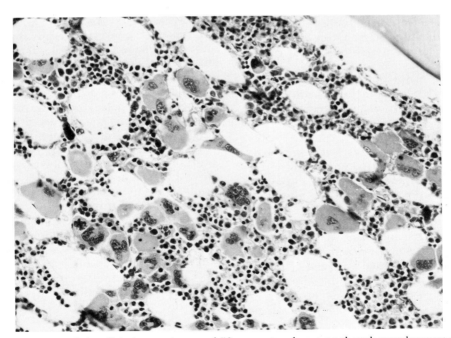

Figure 2–26. Hematopoietic cellularity may be scored 50 per cent or less, even though megakaryocytes are grossly overabundant. The presence of an occasional megakaryocyte in mitosis is not specific for any form of leukemia. 250×, H&E.

of marrow fibrosis analogous to this event in polycythemia vera.[4] Progression to acute leukemia also occurs.[5] Whether this leukemia is myeloblastic or megakaryoblastic has not been convincingly elucidated.

The marrow histopathology of essential thrombocythemia must be distinguished from that of the allied myeloproliferative diseases as well as from reactive thrombocytosis. In polycythemia vera the normoblastic proliferation is generally the dominating feature even when megakaryocytes are overly numerous. When erythropoiesis is depressed in polycythemia vera, however, the number of normoblasts is decreased, and the marrow composition may simulate that of essential thrombocythemia. Red cell mass and plasma volume determinations in a nonbleeding iron-repleted state distinguish the diseases. In chronic granulocytic leukemia the marrow population is dominated by the granulocytic lineage, although the megakaryocytes may be increased in number. Distinction from the uncommon variant of chronic granulocytic leukemia characterized by an unusually high megakaryocytic content is usually possible on the basis of megakaryocytic morphology. In essential thrombocythemia the megakaryocytes, as a rule, are larger and show nuclear complexity, whereas in the variant form of granulocytic leukemia the megakaryocytes are small and have nonlobated nuclei typical of micromegakaryocytes. Confusion between these diseases can usually be resolved by leukocyte alkaline phosphatase determination and chromosome studies. The distinction of the marrow of chronic primary myelofibrosis from that of essential thrombocythemia depends on the presence of collagen fibrosis, with megakaryocyte entrapment in the former and its absence in the latter.

Reactive thrombocytosis with megakaryocytosis can develop in patients with hemorrhage, thrombosis, infection, and cancer. Only rarely is the increase in the number of megakaryocytes more than mild. Relevant studies almost always clarify the diagnosis. Furthermore, the increases in platelets and megakaryocytes subside when these diseases are controlled, whereas in essential thrombocythemia they persist until appropriate chemotherapy is used.

REFERENCES

1. Silverstein, M. N.: Primary thrombocythemia. *In* Williams, W. J., Beutler, E., Erslev, A. J., and Licht-man, M. A. (eds.): Hematology. New York, McGraw-Hill, 1983, pp. 218–221.
2. Pettit, J. E.: Essential thrombocythemia. *In* Hoffbrand, A. V., and Lewis, S. M. (eds.): Postgraduate Haematology. New York, Appleton-Century-Crofts, 1981, pp. 600–603.
3. Harker, L. A., and Finch, C. A.: Thrombokinetics in man. J Clin Invest 48:963–974, 1969.
4. Silverstein, M. N.: Agnogenic Myeloid Metaplasia. Acton, Massachusetts, Publishing Science Group, Inc., 1975, pp. 81–82.
5. Geller, S. A., and Shapiro, E.: Acute leukemia as a natural sequel to primary thrombocythemia. Am J Clin Pathol 77:353–356, 1982.

CHRONIC PRIMARY MYELOFIBROSIS (CHRONIC FIBROGENIC MEGAKARYOCYTIC LEUKEMIA)

An inordinate number of names have been applied to this disease, the more commonly used being myelosclerosis with myeloid metaplasia, agnogenic myeloid metaplasia, and megakaryocytic myelosis.[1] Since 1951, the disease has been classified as a myeloproliferative disorder.[2] The neoplastic character of the disease has been established by demonstrating the clonal replication of the erythrocytic, granulocytic, and megakaryocytic lineages. The fibroblastic proliferation, on the other hand, is not clonal.[3] Thus, the fibrosis, which is an all important feature of the disease, is a reactive fibroplasia rather than a neoplasia. Since platelets contain enzymes and produce a growth factor capable of promoting collagen synthesis, the megakaryocytes or their product platelets may be responsible for the fibrosis.[4–6]

Collagen fibrosis of the marrow can follow in the wake of polycythemia vera or essential thrombocythemia to produce a morphology that can be indistinguishable from chronic primary myelofibrosis. The designations postpolycythemic myelofibrosis and postthrombocythemic myelofibrosis have been applied to this complication. Although the event has been considered to represent a conversion from one myeloproliferative disease to another,[2] the nonclonal character of the fibrosis, the differences between polycythemia vera and essential thrombocythemia in karyotypic lesions, and the differences between the spent phase of polycythemia vera and chronic primary myelofibrosis in erythroid cytokinetics do not support this interpretation.[3, 7, 8]

Marked splenomegaly in the absence of lymph node enlargement and in conjunction with leukoerythroblastosis and tailed poikilocytic red cells in the peripheral blood are characteristic of the disease. Typically the marrow cannot be aspirated.[9, 10] A provisional diagnosis must be substantiated by specific morphology in the marrow. Therefore, the marrow core biopsy is an essential procedure for the diagnosis.

In the marrow megakaryocytes entrapped in collagenized fibrous tissue is the salient feature required for a tenable diagnosis (Figs. 2–27 to 2–30). Characteristically the megakaryocytes are overly abundant, occur singly or in clusters, and commonly show structural abnormalities. These include bizarre cell shape, too few or too many nuclear lobes, and scanty or excessive cytoplasm. As a rule, megakaryocyte morphology is more variable and abnormal than in either polycythemia vera or essential thrombocythemia. When these diseases develop collagen fibrosis, their megakaryocytes are more dysplastic. This is especially evident in and around the fibrotic sites. The collagenized fibrous tissue is variable in quantity. Whether the collagen is focal and limited or sufficiently abundant to occupy most of the intertrabecular space, megakaryocytes are always present in the collagen even if they are diminished in absolute number.

Three subsidiary features complete the principal morphology of the marrow. First, metaplastic bone, when present, can be more or less abundant than the collagen (Fig. 2–31). Second, dilated sinusoids are commonly impinged upon by or contain megakaryocytes and nucleated red cells (Fig. 2–30). Third, marrow hypercellularity when present is usually caused by an increase in granulocytes (Fig. 2–29). When collagen is limited, the hypercellularity is a prominent feature, but when collagen or bone is abundant, the cellularity can be greatly diminished. Fat cells may be present even when collagen and metaplastic bone are abundant.

In the diagnostic considerations it should be recognized that an increase in reticulin in the marrow, "reticulin fibrosis," occurs in many hematological neoplasias and therefore should not be accepted as prima facie evidence of chronic primary myelofibrosis or of postpolycythemic or postthrombocythemic fibrosis.[11–13] Similarly, collagen fibrosis occurs in a variety of marrow diseases, including the blast crisis of chronic granulocytic leukemia, acute leukemia following chemotherapy, granulomatous inflammation, and metastatic carcinoma to the marrow. In megakaryocytic evolution of chronic granulocytic leukemia in which there may be collagen fibrosis, mi-

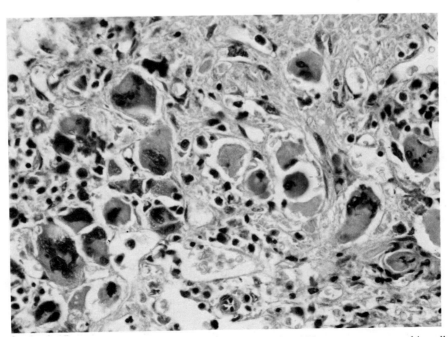

Figure 2–27. Abnormal megakaryocytes, some of which are enlarged and bizarre, are entrapped in collagen fibrous tissue. Even in the smaller megakaryocytes, the apparently nonlobated nuclei are highly irregular and hyperchromatic. The megakaryocytes do not appear compressed by the collagen unless the specimen is subjected to undue compression during biopsy. 400×, H&E.

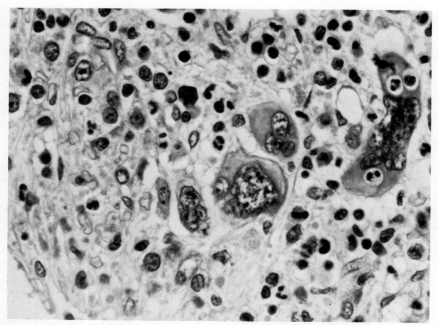

Figure 2–28. A group of large bizarre megakaryocytes in which the nuclear chromatin is chaotically dispersed. One contains granulocytes, which is a feature found in normal as well as abnormal megakaryocytes and called emperipolesis. Not all or even the majority of megakaryocytes need be engulfed in collagen in this disease. 600×, H&E.

cromegakaryocytes rather than large and bizarre megakaryocytes are present. Therefore, the stringent criterion of abnormal megakaryocytes with collagen entrapment should be adhered to in rendering the diagnosis of this disease.

Evolution from chronic primary myelofibrosis and polycythemia vera complicated by

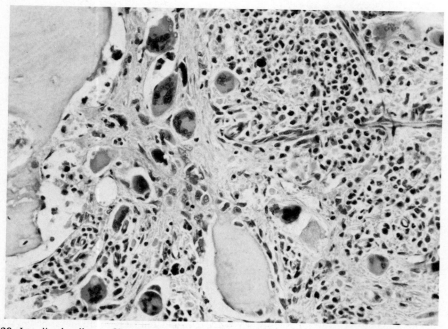

Figure 2–29. Localized collagen fibrosis with megakaryocytic entrapment commonly occurs adjacent to the bone. Frequently the trabecular bone surface is irregular consequent to new bone formation. Occasionally osteoblasts cover the bone surface. The majority of the remaining cells are granulocytes. 250×, H&E.

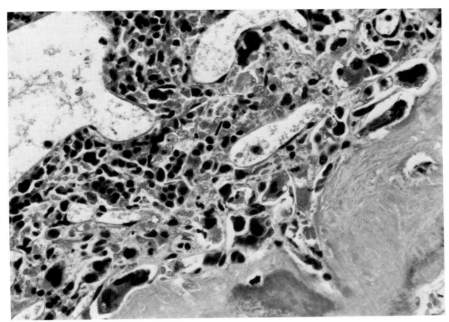

Figure 2–30. In postpolycythemic myelofibrosis, the sinusoids may yet be in a conspicuously dilated state. A megakaryocyte protrudes into one. 400×, H&E.

fibrosis to acute leukemia occurs in about 5 to 15 per cent of cases.[9, 10] Although claimed to be solely of myeloblastic or myelomonocytic morphology, the leukemia can be megakaryoblastic in some instances of chronic primary myelofibrosis.[14, 15]

REFERENCES

1. Ward, H. P., and Block, M. H.: The natural history of agnogenic myeloid metaplasia and a critical evaluation of its relationship with the myeloproliferative syndrome. Medicine 50:357–420, 1971.

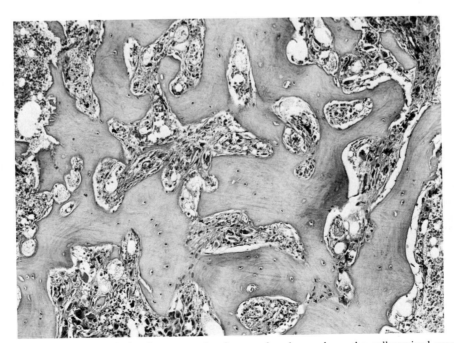

Figure 2–31. A complex labyrinth of anastomosing bone trabeculae encloses the collagenized marrow with its bizarre imprisoned megakaryocytes. This degree of bone formation is uncommon. 100×, H&E.

2. Dameshak, W.: Some speculations on the myeloproliferative syndrome. Blood 6:372–375, 1951.

3. Jacobson, R. J., Salo, A., and Fialkow, P. J.: Agnogenic myeloid metaplasia: A clonal proliferation of hematopoietic stem cells with secondary myelofibrosis. Blood 51:189–194, 1978.

4. Anttinen, H., Tuderman, L., Oikarinen, A., et al.: Intracellular enzymes of collagen biosynthesis in human platelets. Blood 50:29–37, 1977.

5. Groopman, J. E.: The pathogenesis of myelofibrosis in myeloproliferative disorders. Ann Intern Med 92:857–858, 1980.

6. Castro-Malaspina, H., Rabellino, E. M., Yen, A., et al.: Human megakaryocyte stimulation of proliferation of bone marrow fibroblasts. Blood 57:781–787, 1981.

7. Rowley, J. D.: Cytogenetic studies in hematologic disorders. In Hoffband, A. V. (ed.): Recent Advances in Haematology. Edinburgh, Churchill Livingstone, 1982, pp. 233–252.

8. Kornberg, A., Fibach, E., Treves, A., et al.: Circulating erythroid progenitors in patients with "spent" polycythaemia vera and myelofibrosis with myeloid metaplasia. Br J Haematol 52:573–578, 1982.

9. Silverstein, M. N.: Agnogenic myeloid metaplasia. In Williams, W. J., Beutler, E., Erslev, A. J., and Lichtman, M. A. (eds.): Hematology. New York, McGraw-Hill, 1983, pp. 214–218.

10. Silverstein, M. N.: Agnogenic Myeloid Metaplasia. Acton, Massachusetts, Publishing Science Group, Inc., 1975.

11. Burston, J., and Pinniger, J. L.: The reticulin content of bone marrow in haematological disorders. Br J Haematol 9:172–184, 1963.

12. Sanerkin, N. G.: Stromal changes in leukaemic and related bone marrow proliferation. J Clin Pathol 17:541–547, 1964.

13. Roberts, B. E., Miles, D. W., and Woods, C. G.: Polycythaemia vera and myelosclerosis: A bone marrow study. Br J Haematol 16:75–85, 1969.

14. Breton-Gorius, J., Daniel, M. T., Flandrin, G., et al.: Fine structure and peroxidase activity of circulating micromegakaryoblasts and platelets in a case of acute myelofibrosis. Br J Haematol 25:331–339, 1973.

15. Efrati, P., Nir, E., Yaari, A., et al.: Myeloproliferative disorders terminating in acute micromegakaryoblastic leukemia. Br J Haematol 43:79–86, 1979.

MYELOSCLEROSIS WITH MYELOID METAPLASIA: A REVISED VIEW

The introduction of the concept of the myeloproliferative syndrome by Dameshek in 1951 solidified attention on the kinship of the chronic hematopoietic diseases known as chronic granulocytic leukemia, polycythemia vera, essential thrombocythemia, and myelosclerosis with myeloid metaplasia.[1] Basic tenets upon which the concept rested included the suppositions that (1) all of these diseases were malignant neoplasias, (2) intermediate forms existed in which manifestations of two or even three of the diseases could be displayed concurrently, and (3) complete conversions or transformations occurred between the disease entities. In clearly declared cases of each disease, normoblastic, granulocytic, megakaryocytic, or fibroblastic lineages prevailed, but lineal preponderance could wane or completely change.

In recent years, cytogenetic studies initially and isoenzyme analysis subsequently have provided strong support for the neoplastic nature of all the cell replications involved in these diseases with the notable exception of the marrow fibroblast or stromal cell.[2] By inference, therefore, the marrow fibroplasia or myelosclerosis can be considered nonneoplastic and to merely coexist with and possibly be induced by the neoplastic hematopoietic cells. Ample precedent exists for this conclusion; there are many examples of cancer-associated reactive fibrosis in and outside the bone marrow. While these data essentially resolve the disputed neoplastic status concerning some of these diseases, notably polycythemia vera and myelosclerosis with myeloid metaplasia,[3] and demonstrate the reactive character of the fibrosis, they create the problem of interpreting cases in which marrow fibroplasia or myelosclerosis occurs initially or develops later in the course of the clinical disease.

The bone marrow in man normally contains only a few scattered reticulin fibers, and collagen is limited to thin perivascular collars.* A wide variety of reactions or diseases affecting the marrow serve to provoke an increase of the reticulin fibers.[4, 5] These range from compensatory hyperplasias to acute and chronic leukemias and lymphomas and from granulomatous inflammation to metastatic cancer. This so-called "reticulin fibrosis" need not be permanent. It can recede and disappear with removal of the stimulus. A dramatic demonstration of this reversal occurs in treated acute or chronic leukemia.[6, 7] On the other hand, progression from reticular fibrosis to collagen fibrosis may occur. A

---

*The difference between reticulin and collagen appears to be largely quantitative rather than qualitative, since the essential biochemical and ultrastructural properties of reticulin are those of collagen. The argyrophilic reticulin fibers are probably transformed into tinctorial collagen fibers by coalescence of neighboring fibers or by accretion of molecular collagen onto the reticulin fibers with consequent loss or inaccessibility of the silver binding groups. Nonetheless, and although artificial, the distinction between the two fibers is sanctioned by practice and is useful in the present context.

classic example is the development of collagen fibrosis in cases of polycythemia vera. This event has been interpreted as a conversion of polycythemia vera to myelosclerosis with myeloid metaplasia.[8, 9] The recent demonstration of a striking difference between spent polycythemia vera and myelosclerosis with myeloid metaplasia in erythropoietin dependency of the cytokinetic response in vitro argues strongly against this view.[10] Similarly, the development of collagen fibrosis has been emphasized in chronic granulocytic leukemia and acute myeloblastic leukemia and has led to similar claims of transitional states or transformation to myelosclerosis.[11, 12] The current evidence of distinctive chromosomal lesions in these diseases and of a fibroblastic proliferation that is reactive rather than neoplastic is likewise contrary to such conclusions. Moreover, the postulated kinship of these diseases based on a single multipotential cell capable of producing fibroblasts as well as hematopoietic cells is no longer tenable.[13]

Myelosclerosis with myeloid metaplasia appeared as a disease entity in the medical literature approximately 100 years ago.[8] The diversity of views expressed concerning its etiology and pathogenesis during the past century is ably reflected by the array of names given to the disease.[3, 14] Some of the views advocated that the disorder is a form of leukemia and promoted the role of the megakaryocyte as the culprit cell. This idea was based on the observation in some cases of a prodigious increase in the number of megakaryocytes, many highly atypical, and of the persistence of these cells within expanses of collagen despite the depletion of red cell and granulocyte precursors from the marrow. That the megakaryocyte or its blast precursor may be the prevailing cell in a leukemia, in a role analogous to that of the granulocyte and the red cell, and that this occurs more frequently than was recognized previously is suggested by two recent advances: (1) the specific identification of circulating blasts as megakaryoblasts in some leukemias[15–18] and (2) the delineation of the disease acute myelosclerosis and its subsequent recognition as acute megakaryoblastic leukemia.[19, 20] Furthermore, the acute leukemia developing in cases of agnogenic myelofibrosis with myeloid metaplasia has been shown to be a leukemia of megakaryoblasts.[15, 21] These observations are in accord with the evidence that the megakaryocyte in myelosclerosis with myeloid metaplasia is neoplastic.[22]

Recently two clues have appeared to provide a link between the megakaryocyte and collagen and bone formation. First, the α-granule of platelets secretes a growth factor capable of stimulating fibroblast replication and collagen and bone synthesis.[23–25] This factor also occurs in megakaryocytes.[26] Second, platelets contain enzymes necessary to catalyze collagen synthesis.[27] While normally both serve physiological functions in hemostasis and repair, under certain conditions they may also promote pathology. Such pathologic events appear to be exemplified by the accumulation of abnormal neoplastic megakaryocytes and their product platelets in the marrow in association with collagen fibrosis and bone formation in cases of myelosclerosis with myeloid metaplasia, polycythemia vera, essential thrombocythemia, and chronic granulocytic leukemia with a high content of micromegakaryocytes. Undoubtedly other pathogenetic mechanisms for marrow fibrosis exist; in these chronic leukemias the neoplastic megakaryocyte appears to occupy the pivotal role.

At some time in these chronic leukemias myeloid metaplasia may occur. Extramedullary hematopoiesis, also known as myeloid metaplasia, is defined as the presence of red cell, granulocyte, or platelet precursors at sites other than the marrow. The former term is preferred since the latter implies that all of the cells originate at the site of replication and maturation. Extramedullary hematopoiesis is not restricted to leukemias; it also occurs in chronic hemolytic anemias and in other states of intense blood cell demand. The usual locations of extramedullary hematopoiesis are the spleen, the liver, and the lymph nodes. The predilection for and apparent development in these sites has been rationalized by invoking their hematopoietic potential during fetal life.[3] Accumulated experimental data extending from the basic observations of Till and McCulloch[28] to those more recently obtained,[29, 30] however, support a more tenable and testable thesis—namely, that splenic hematopoiesis is produced by marrow-derived cells that have escaped prematurely into the blood stream consequent to medullary sinusoidal damage mediated by a collagenase.[31] Cytokinetic data[32] and morphological and biochemical studies on megakaryocytes and platelets[33] suggest that an analogous mechanism is operative in humans. Furthermore, there is no compelling evidence that in these chronic leukemias hematopoietic precursors do not metastasize from the marrow to sites of extramedullary hematopoiesis and continue to replicate, differentiate, and mature. Metastatic dissemination is acknowledged for virtually all other types of cancer, and preferential sites of deposition are the rule.

In conclusion, the two morphologic features of myelosclerosis with myeloid metaplasia, marrow fibrosis and extramedullary hematopoiesis, can occur singly or in combination, simultaneously or sequentially. They can develop in many different diseases, whether neoplastic or nonneoplastic, leukemic or nonleukemic. The diversity of these circumstances suggests that myelofibrosis with myeloid metaplasia might be viewed better as a syndrome of multiple etiologies and pathogenetic mechanisms rather than as a disease entity. In the myeloproliferative diseases current evidence indicates that the fibroplasia is reactive rather than neoplastic, occurs as reticulin or collagen, and develops indiscriminately in these as well as other leukemias. The megakaryocytic and platelet α-granule with its fibroblast growth factor and a collagenase may have critical roles in chronic primary myelofibrosis by inducing fibrosis and impairing sinusoidal integrity. The extramedullary hematopoiesis could then occur by metastasis although origin in situ may also be possible. When these complications occur in polycythemia vera, essential thrombocythemia, and chronic granulocytic leukemia with a high content of micromegakaryocytes they could have the same or a similar pathogenesis.

Among the many recorded cases of myelosclerosis with myeloid metaplasia are some that by current criteria can be designated more properly by the term chronic fibrogenic megakaryocytic leukemia rather than as chronic primary myelofibrosis. Many of the other cases represent polycythemia vera, essential thrombocythemia, or chronic granulocytic leukemia complicated by marrow fibrosis. Still others are a variety of diseases, including granulomatous inflammations and metastatic carcinoma and sarcoma. The understanding of acute myelosclerosis has followed an analogous but more rapid evolution. This disease is now recognized as an acute form of megakaryocytic or megakaryoblastic leukemia to be clearly distinguished from masquerading cases of acute myeloblastic or lymphoblastic leukemia with reactive fibrosis. Replacement of the term myelosclerosis with myeloid metaplasia and its numerous synonyms by specific diagnoses is feasible by current methodology and is necessary if specific therapy is to be applied.

REFERENCES

1. Dameshek, W.: Some speculations on the myeloproliferative syndrome. Blood 6:372–375, 1951.
2. Adamson, J. W., and Fialkow, P. J.: The pathogenesis of myeloproliferative syndromes. Br J Haematol 38:299–303, 1978.
3. Ward, H. P., and Block, M. H.: The natural history of agnogenic myeloid metaplasia and a critical evaluation of its relationship with the myeloproliferative syndrome. Medicine 50:357–420, 1971.
4. Burston, J., and Pinniger, J. L.: The reticulin content of bone marrow in haematological disorders. Br J Haematol 9:172–184, 1963.
5. Sanerkin, N. G.: Stromal changes in leukemia and related bone marrow proliferations. J Clin Pathol 17:541–547, 1964.
6. Wittels, B.: Bone marrow biopsy changes following chemotherapy for acute leukemia. Am J Surg Pathol 4:135–142, 1980.
7. McGlave, P. G., Brunning, R. D., Hurd, D. D., et al.: Reversal of severe bone marrow fibrosis and osteosclerosis following allogenic bone marrow transplantation for chronic granulocytic leukemia. Br J Haematol 52:189–194, 1982.
8. Gunz, F., and Baikie, A. G.: Leukemia. New York, Grune & Stratton, 1974, pp. 377–430.
9. Modan, B.: Inter-relationship between polycythaemia vera, leukaemia and myeloid metaplasia. Clin Haematol 4:427–439, 1975.
10. Kornberg, A., Fibach, E., Treves, A., et al.: Circulating erythroid progenitors in patients with "spent" polycythaemia vera and myelofibrosis with myeloid metaplasia. Br J Haematol 52:572–578, 1982.
11. Krauss, S.: Chronic myelocytic leukemia with features simulating myelofibrosis with myeloid metaplasia. Cancer 19:1321–1332, 1966.
12. Lubin, J., Rozen, S., and Rywlin, A.: Malignant myelosclerosis. Arch Intern Med 136:141–145, 1976.
13. Hutt, M. S. R., Pinniger, J. L., and Wetherley-Mein, G.: The myeloproliferative disorders with special reference to myelofibrosis. Blood 8:295–314, 1953.
14. Rappaport, H.: Tumors of the Hematopoietic System. Washington, D.C., Armed Forces Institute of Pathology, 1966, pp. 312–336.
15. Breton-Gorius, J., Daniel, M. T., Flandrin, G., et al.: Fine structure and peroxidase activity of circulating micromegakaryoblasts and platelets in a case of acute myelofibrosis. Br J Haematol 25:331–339, 1973.
16. Breton-Gorius, J., Reyes, F., Duhamel, G., et al.: Megakaryoblastic acute leukemia: Identification by the ultrastructural demonstration of platelet peroxidase. Blood 51:45–60, 1978.
17. Marie, J. P., Vernant, J. P., Dreyfus, B., et al.: Ultrastructural localization of peroxidases in undifferentiated blasts during the blast crisis of chronic granulocytic leukemia. Br J Haematol 43:549–558, 1979.
18. Bevan, D., Rose, M., and Greaves, M.: Leukaemia

of platelet precursors: Diverse features in four cases. Br J Haematol 51:147–164, 1982.

19. den Ottolander, G. J., te Velde, J., Brederoo, P., et al.: Megakaryoblastic leukaemia (acute myelofibrosis): A report of three cases. Br J Haematol 42:9–20, 1979.

20. Bain, B. J., Catovsky, D., O'Brien, M., et al.: Megakaryoblastic leukemia presenting as acute myelofibrosis—a study of four cases with the platelet-peroxidase reaction. Blood 58:206–213, 1981.

21. Efrati, P., Nir, E., Yaari, A., et al.: Myeloproliferative disorders terminating in acute micromegakaryoblastic leukemia. Br J Haematol 43:79–86, 1979.

22. Jacobson, R. J., Salo, A., and Fialkow, P. J.: Agnogenic myeloid metaplasia: A clonal proliferation of hematopoietic stem cells with secondary myelofibrosis. Blood 51:189–194, 1978.

23. Groopman, J. E.: The pathogenesis of myelofibrosis in myeloproliferative disorders. Ann Intern Med 92:857–858, 1980.

24. Moore, M. A. S.: Bone marrow culture: Leucopoiesis and stem cells. *In* Hoffbrand, A. V. (ed.): Recent Advances in Haematology. Edinburgh, Churchill Livingstone, 1982, pp. 136–142.

25. Canalis, E.: Effect of platelet-derived growth factor on DNA and protein synthesis in cultured rat calvaria. Metabolism 30:970–975, 1981.

26. Castro-Malaspina, H., Rabellino, E. M., Yen, A., et al.: Human megakaryocytic stimulation of proliferation of bone marrow fibroblasts. Blood 57:781–787, 1981.

27. Anttinen, H., Tuderman, L., Oikarinen, A., et al.: Intracellular enzymes of collagen biosynthesis in human platelets. Blood 50:29–37, 1977.

28. Till, J. E., and McCulloch, E. A.: A direct measurement of the radiation sensitivity of normal mouse bone marrow. Radiat Res 14:213–222, 1961.

29. Rencricca, N. J., Rizzoli, V., Howard, D., et al.: Stem cell migration and proliferation during severe anemia. Blood 36:764–771, 1970.

30. Wang, J. C., and Tobin, M. S.: Mechanism of extramedullary haematopoiesis in rabbits with saponin-induced myelofibrosis and myeloid metaplasia. Br J Haematol 51:277–284, 1982.

31. Cherney, C. M., Harper, E., and Colmans, R. W.: Human platelet collagenase. J Clin Invest 53:1647–1654, 1974.

32. Wang, J. C., Cheung, C. P., Ahmed, F., et al.: Circulating granulocyte and macrophage progenitor cells in primary and secondary myelofibrosis. Br J Haematol 54:301–307, 1983.

33. Breton-Gorius, J., Bizet, M., Reyes, F., et al.: Myelofibrosis and acute megakaryoblastic leukemia in a child: Topographic relationship between fibroblasts and megakaryocytes with an α-granule defect. Leuk Res 6:97–110, 1982.

MYELODYSPLASIA

The French-American-British Cooperative Group has recently advocated a revised definition and classification of hematopoietic cell maturation defects in which the morphological abnormalities are insufficient for a diagnosis of leukemia.[1] The term "myelodysplasia" has been applied to these atypical or deranged maturations. This designation is preferable to such terminology as smoldering leukemia, preleukemia, and oligoblastic leukemia because these terms imply impending or actual acute leukemia, and many cases do not progress to or terminate in unequivocal acute leukemia. Precedence for the view connoted by the term dysplasia can be found in many epithelial cell maturation abnormalities, one of the most thoroughly studied being squamous cell carcinoma of the uterine cervix; some cases of cervical dysplasia progress to carcinoma, some remain stable, and some remit.

In their latest publication, the FAB group proposed a classification of myelodysplasia with five defined types: (1) refractory anemia, (2) refractory anemia with ring sideroblasts, (3) refractory anemia with excess blast cells, (4) refractory anemia with excess blast cells in transformation, and (5) chronic myelomonocytic disorder.

Patients with these disorders are most frequently over 50 years old. Splenomegaly is uncommon. Anemia that has an undefinable etiology and that is unresponsive to standard therapy is an almost invariable feature. The morphology of the anemia and some of its functional characteristics have been described in detail, as have the frequently associated abnormalities of the white cells and platelets.[2,3]

The marrow core biopsy is most useful in assessing the quantitative aspects and some of the qualitative features in these disorders. Only in conjunction with other studies, however, can the core specimen be used to derive a definitive diagnosis.[4-6] Although maturational defects can theoretically involve one, two, or all three of the myeloid lineages simultaneously, thereby allowing any one of seven possible permutations of myelodysplasia to develop, the abnormalities are usually most evident in two of the cell lines; for example, megakaryocytes in combination with normoblasts or megakaryocytes with granulocytes.

In the refractory anemias the marrow cellularity is normal or increased to as much as 100 per cent. It is rarely decreased. The most arresting features are in the erythroid and megakaryocytic series (Fig. 2–32). Nucleated red cells are predominant, and there is an obviously disproportionate increase of the early forms—erythroblasts and basophilic and polychromatophilic normoblasts. In this respect the features mimic megaloblastosis of vitamin B_{12} and folate deficiency and erythroleukemia. Study of marrow smear prepa-

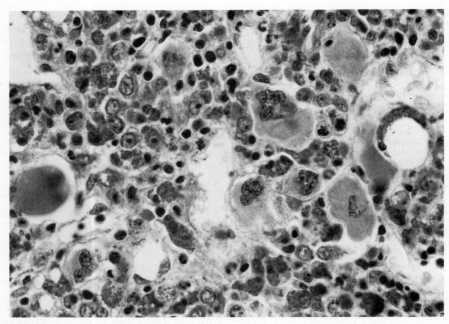

Figure 2–32. Refractory anemia with ring sideroblasts in a 66-year-old man with marked anemia, reticulocytopenia, and neutropenia. The marrow is moderately hypercellular, red cell maturation is impaired as indicated by an increase in erythroblasts and early normoblasts, and megakaryocytes are moderately increased in number and slightly atypical. These are numerous hemosiderin-laden histiocytes. 520×, H&E.

rations is necessary for detection of detailed nuclear and cytoplasmic abnormalities and the telltale siderotic rings. Usually megakaryocyte abnormalities are as conspicuous as the faulty erythroid maturation. The megakaryocytes are commonly slightly to moderately increased in number but rarely to the degree obtained in the megakaryocytic leukemias or in chronic granulocytic leukemia with a high content of micromegakaryocytes. The cells are variable in size and contour, with many being small. Nuclear aberrations are common and include hypo- or hyperlobation, marked variations in size, shape, and chromicity, and peculiarities in lobe distribution (Figs. 2–32 to 2–34). Mitoses may be present. Granulocyte abnormalities, if present, are evident as a decrease in mature forms (Fig. 2–34). In the refractory anemias with or without ring sideroblasts, myelocytes may be disproportionately abundant, but by definition blast cells are less than 5 per cent of the granulocyte-monocyte lineage. On the other hand, in the refractory anemias with excess blast cells or in transformation, the number of myeloblasts is increased. By current standards myeloblasts and promyelocytes must be less than 30 per cent of the hematopoietic cell population of the marrow in myelodysplasia. Cases with a greater percentage are considered leukemia.

In contrast to the refractory anemias in which erythroid cells dominate the marrow pathology, in the chronic myelomonocytic disorder the granulocytes, monocytes, or both prevail. In the most readily identifiable cases there is an obvious increase in the number of myelocytes or monocytes, or both, that is associated with a slight increase in myeloblasts and an obvious decrease in mature granulocytes (Figs. 2–34 and 2–35). Qualitative abnormalities of the erythroid and megakaryocytic lines, if present, are those of the refractory anemias.

Hemosiderin may be increased, sometimes markedly, related to failure to utilize iron and to repetitive blood transfusion. Reticulin is usually increased but collagen is not present.

In the differential diagnosis the distinction from the vitamin-dependent maturational defects and from acute myeloblastic leukemia, erythroleukemia, and megakaryocytic leukemia is most important. In the former standard assays and therapeutic trials of B_{12}, folate, and pyridoxine are used, whereas in the latter careful and critical analysis of the marrow usually resolves the problem. Distinction between the exact type of refractory anemia is of secondary importance. For the chronic myelomonocytic disorder uncertainties may arise from similarities with chronic

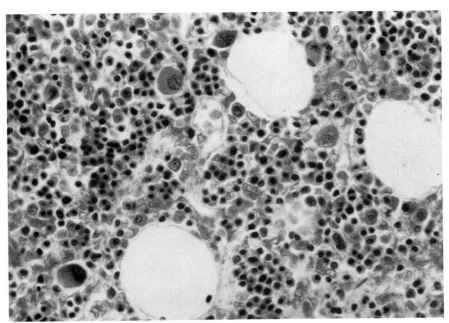

Figure 2–33. Pancytopenia in an 82-year-old woman whose marrow is moderately hypercellular. The principal features are the micromegakaryocytes, the erythroid predominance, the increase in hemosiderin, and the dearth of granulocytes. 400×, H&E.

myelomonocytic or granulocytic leukemia. The distinction from the former condition is unclear currently, but the presence of the Philadelphia chromosomal defect would be definitive evidence for the latter. In the past some cases of myelodysplasia have been designated as malignant or acute myelosclerosis. These terms should be abandoned.

The evolution of myelodysplasia is variable. Some cases develop abruptly and termi-

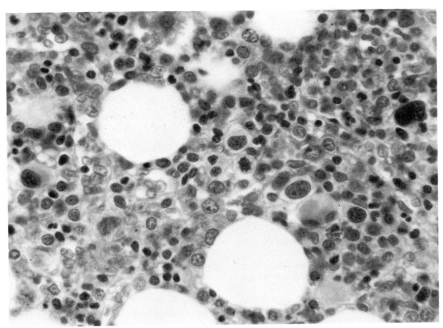

Figure 2–34. Refractory anemia with excess blast cells in a woman who had moderate anemia and reticulocytopenia for 14 years. Levels of serum B_{12} and folate were normal and that of iron was elevated. The normocellular marrow contains megakaryocytes with large nonlobated nuclei, 10 to 15 per cent myeloblasts, and decreased numbers of maturing granulocytes and normoblasts. 520×, H&E.

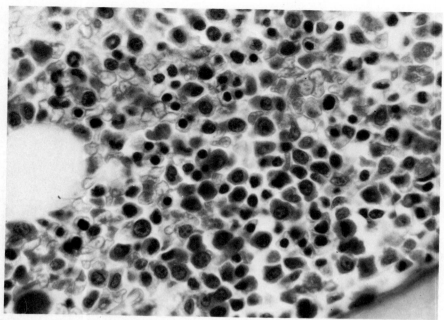

Figure 2–35. A chronic myelomonocytic disorder in a 76-year-old woman with pancytopenia including marked neutropenia. The most prominent feature in the moderately hypercellular marrow is the increase in myelocytes admixed with a few promyelocytes and blast cells. The numbers of megakaryocytes, normoblasts, and mature granulocytes are diminished. The distinction between this form of myelodysplasia and chronic myelomonocytic leukemia is difficult to make. 680×, H&E.

nate in acute leukemia within a year.[4–6] Most cases progress gradually, and a few continue for many years. Approximately 25 per cent lead to acute myeloblastic leukemia.[3]

Myelodysplasia developing several years after chemotherapy or radiation for cancer appears to have the same features and follows a course similar to that of idiopathic cases.[7–9]

REFERENCES

1. Bennett, J. M., Catovsky, D., Daniel, M. T., et al.: Proposals for the classification of the myelodysplastic syndromes. Br J Haematol 51:189–199, 1982.
2. Linman, J. W., and Bagby, G. C.: The preleukemic syndrome. Cancer 42:854–864, 1978.
3. Weber, R. F. A., Geraedts, J. P. M., Kerkhof, H., et al.: The preleukemic syndrome. Acta Med Scand 207:391–395, 1980.
4. Bennett, J. M., Catovsky, D., Daniel, M. T., et al.: Proposals for the classification of the acute leukaemias. Br J Haematol 33:451–458, 1976.
5. Gralnick, H. R., Galton, D. A. G., Catovsky, D., et al.: Classification of acute leukemia. Ann Intern Med 87:740–753, 1977.
6. Bennett, J. M.: The French-American-British classification of the acute adult myeloid leukemias. *In* Bloomfield, C. D. (ed.): Acute Leukemia. The Hague, Martinus Nijhoff, 1982, pp. 109–125.
7. Vardiman, J. W., Golomb, H. M., Rowley, J. D., et al.: Acute nonlymphocytic leukemia in malignant lymphoma. Cancer 42:229–242, 1978.
8. Foucar, K., McKenna, R. W., Bloomfield, C. D., et al.: Therapy-related leukemia. Cancer 43:1285–1296, 1979.
9. Sultan, C., Sigaux, F., Imbert, M., et al.: Acute myelodysplasia with myelofibrosis: A report of eight cases. Br J Haematol 49:11–16, 1981.

TREATED ACUTE LEUKEMIA

Currently patients with acute leukemia or chronic granulocytic leukemia progressing to blast cell crisis, with few exceptions, are treated with myelosuppressive or myelotoxic drugs. Although examination of aspirated marrow is usually satisfactory to establish the diagnosis, the marrow core specimen has proved to be superior for intra- or posttherapy evaluation. The reasons for this are that (1) the core permits more accurate quantitative and qualitative comparisons; (2) during or after therapy the marrow is frequently too hypocellular to yield an adequate sample by aspiration; and (3) collagen fibrosis may develop and prevent aspiration. Familiarity with the histopathology of the marrow after chemotherapy is therefore essential for assessing the adequacy of treatment.

The changes in the marrow after chemotherapy can be considered as occurring in

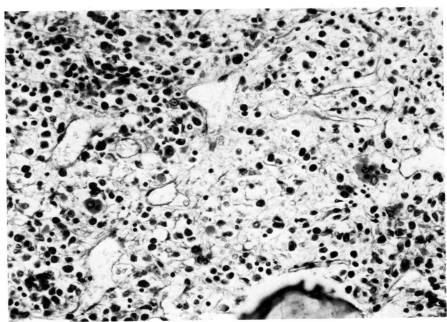

Figure 2–36. Acute myeloblastic leukemia approximately ten days after initiation of chemotherapy. There is focal depletion of the marrow. 250×, H&E.

two overlapping sequential phases, cellular depletion and marrow reconstitution.[1] In the marrow core specimen focal hypocellularity is the first morphological indication of effective therapy (Fig. 2–36). Cell loss is progressive, but total depletion may require a month more or less, depending on the particular therapeutic schedule and the sensitivity of the leukemic cells. The mechanism of leukemic cell destruction is not evident morphologically. Extensive necrosis is unusual.

With the emptying of the marrow the stromal reticulin that is increased becomes obvious (Figs. 2–37 and 2–38).[2] Since reticu-

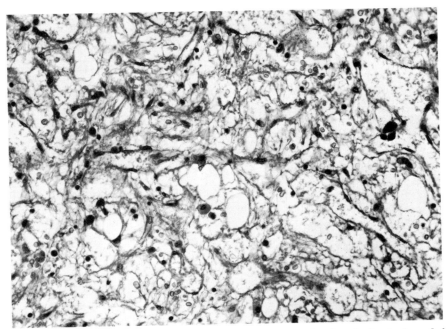

Figure 2–37. Chronic granulocytic leukemia in blast cell crisis three weeks after the beginning of chemotherapy. The marrow space is filled by an essentially empty fibrillar web carrying a few dilated sinusoids. 250×, H&E.

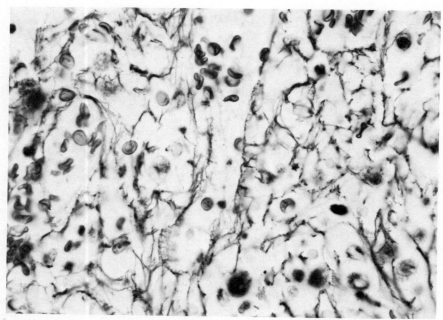

Figure 2–38. Acute myeloblastic leukemia following reinduction chemotherapy after relapse. The stain for reticulin shows the character and abundance of the fibrils in the cell-depleted marrow space. 680×, Wilder.

lin is substantially increased in many hematopoietic neoplasias,[3] the increase cannot be attributed to the therapy. Scattered throughout the stroma are many dilated sinusoids containing fibrin. Focal hemorrhage is common. Despite the effectiveness of the drugs, well-preserved mature plasma cells remain, usually aligned along small blood vessels (Fig. 2–39). Small clusters of well-differentiated lymphocytes are also frequently present.

As leukemic depletion progresses and approaches its maximum, fat cell generation develops, followed by a repopulation of the marrow by megakaryocytes, normoblasts,

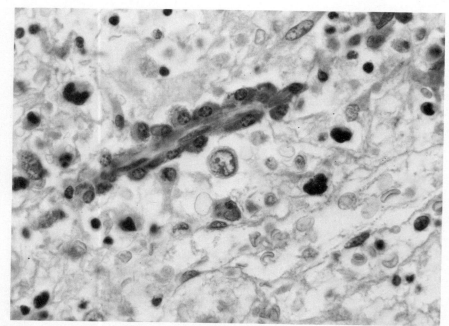

Figure 2–39. Acute myeloblastic leukemia following reinduction chemotherapy after relapse. Mature plasma cells clinging to a small vessel appear resistant to the cytotoxic drugs used. 680×, H&E.

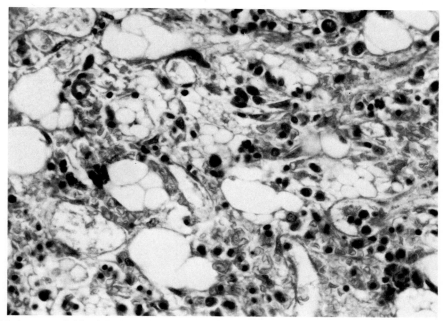

Figure 2–40. Acute myeloblastic leukemia three weeks after induction chemotherapy. Hematopoiesis is accompanied by fat cell generation in the early stages of marrow reconstitution. 400×, H&E.

and granulocytes (Figs. 2–40 and 2–41). Repopulation by the first two usually precedes the appearance of granulocytes. Typically the marrow in therapeutic remission comprises fat cells filling 50 to 90 per cent of the marrow, clusters of normoblasts, mostly orthochromic forms, developing and mature granulocytes, and megakaryocytes, occurring singly or in small clusters. The stromal reticulin decreases and becomes normal in quantity as reconstitution proceeds (Fig. 2–42).[1, 2]

The events in marrow reconstitution after chemotherapy followed by autografting reportedly differ from those occurring in un-

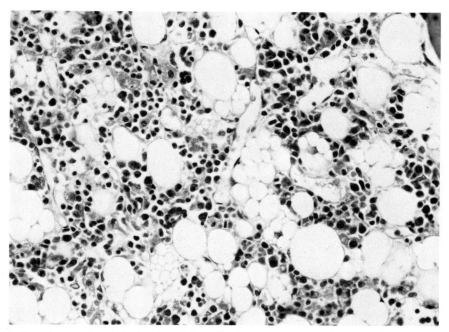

Figure 2–41. Chronic granulocytic leukemia in blast cell crisis approximately five weeks after chemotherapy. The marrow space is replenished by restorative hematopoiesis and fat cell generation. 250×, H&E.

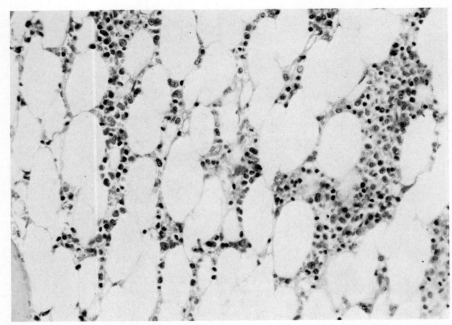

Figure 2–42. Acute myeloblastic leukemia in remission. Based on an expected hematopoietic cell to fat cell ratio of 1 in adults, this marrow is judged as moderately hypocellular, but qualitatively it approximates normalcy. 250×, H&E.

assisted hematopoietic cell regeneration.[4] With grafting, monotypic rather than mixed colonies of normoblasts, granulocytes, or megakaryocytes develop, and these precede fat cell generation.

Whereas in the majority of cases the stromal (reticular) cells are converted to fat cells, in a minority the stromal cells evince fibroblastic properties and produce collagen.[5] The latter response develops more commonly following chemotherapy of chronic granulocytic leukemia or its blast crisis than in acute leukemia. The fibrosis can be focal or widespread and may be accompanied by

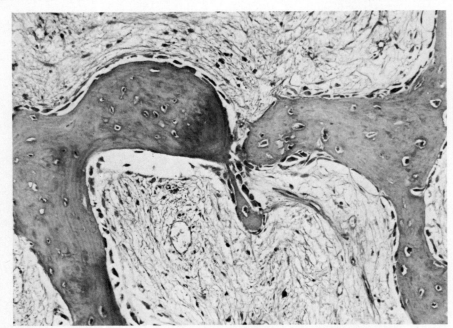

Figure 2–43. Acute myeloblastic leukemia following induction and consolidation chemotherapy. Woven bone formation accompanies widespread fibrosis in the marrow space. 100×, H&E.

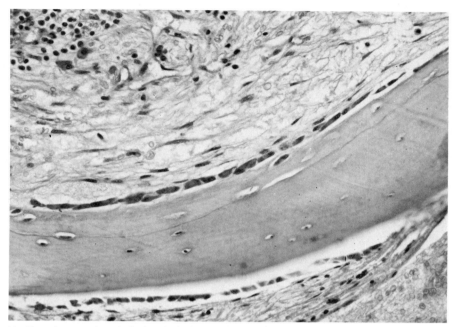

Figure 2–44. Chronic granulocytic leukemia in blast cell crisis after a second course of induction chemotherapy. There is laminar bone formation with the fibrosis in the marrow space. 250×, H&E.

woven or lamellar bone formation (Figs. 2–43 and 2–44). In an occasional instance when leukemic cell depletion is advanced and fat cell generation is present focal serous atrophy of the fat develops (Fig. 2–45).

Excessive numbers of hemosiderin-laden macrophages frequently accumulate. This ac-

cumulation reflects the inadequate iron utilization consequent to decreased normoblast production incident to the leukemia and its therapy. Occasionally bulky macrophages lacking any visible phagocytized material are present (Fig. 2–46) and rarely macrophages form clusters of finely vacuolated foam cells

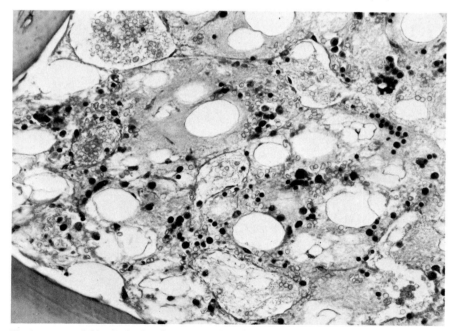

Figure 2–45. Acute myeloblastic leukemia two weeks after completion of induction chemotherapy. Limited hematopoiesis with fat cell generation is associated with focal serous atrophy of fat. 250×, H&E.

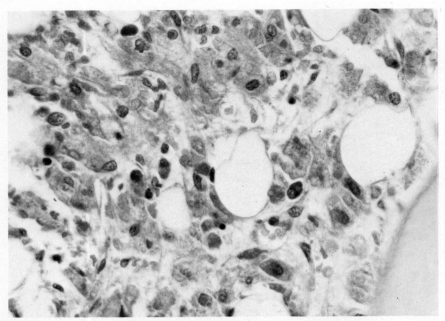

Figure 2–46. Acute myelomonocytic leukemia three weeks after the beginning of induction chemotherapy. Shortly thereafter, the patient died after gastrointestinal hemorrhage, respiratory distress, and renal failure. The marrow space is extensively filled with bulky bland-appearing histiocytes. No cellular phagocytosis is present. Histiocyte proliferation after chemotherapy for acute leukemia has been related to complicating virus infection. 520×, H&E.

that simulate the Niemann-Pick cell (Fig. 2–47). The latter differ from the macrophages that form lipogranulomas.

Of the many profound changes occurring in the marrow as a result of chemotherapy, the two features requiring the most critical evaluation are (1) the number of residual blast cells present (Figs. 2–48 and 2–49) and (2) the number and lineage of maturing hematopoietic cells during recovery. A semi-

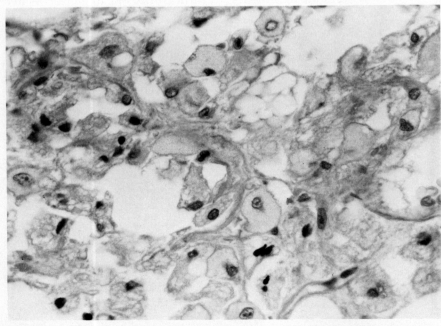

Figure 2–47. Myelodysplasia with excess blast cells progressing to erythroleukemia six weeks after chemotherapy. Small clusters of histiocytes with finely vacuolated cytoplasm are present in the interstices of the fat cells, which extensively fill the marrow. There was no evidence for hyperlipidemia. 520×, H&E.

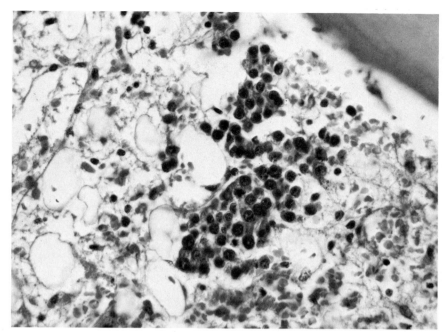

Figure 2—48. Acute myelomonocytic leukemia after reinduction chemotherapy for relapse approximately two years after the initial diagnosis. An isolated focus of blast cells remains in marrow that is otherwise extensively depleted of hematopoietic cells. 400×, H&E.

quantitative estimate is almost always sufficient. According to current standards blast cells can constitute no more than 5 per cent of the hematopoietic cell population in order to declare a state of therapeutic remission.

In an occasional case of the acute myeloid leukemias a postchemotherapy biopsy specimen contains in excess of 5 per cent blast cells and promyelocytes admixed with about an equal number of myelocytes but with few if any more mature forms. Islands of normoblasts and megakaryocytes are also pres-

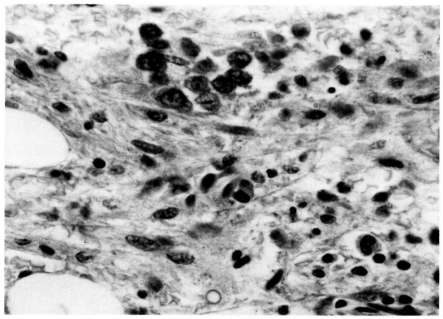

Figure 2—49. Acute myeloblastic leukemia two weeks after initiation of chemotherapy for leukemia that developed after prolonged chlorambucil treatment for metastatic ovarian carcinoma. The marrow shows extensive fibroplasia with a small cluster of entrapped blast cells. 680×, H&E.

ent, as may be regenerating fat cells. The problem of whether the blast cells represent residual leukemia or early marrow reconstitution is best resolved by withholding additional therapy and obtaining another specimen five to ten days later.

REFERENCES

1. Wittels, B.: Bone marrow biopsy changes following chemotherapy for acute leukemia. Am J Surg Pathol 4:135–142, 1980.
2. Manoharan, A., Horsley, R., and Pitney, W. R.: The reticulin content of bone marrow in acute leukemia in adults. Br J Haematol 43:185–190, 1979.
3. Sanerkin, N. G.: Stromal changes in leukemic and related bone marrow proliferations. J Clin Pathol 17:541–547, 1964.
4. Islam, A., Catovsky, D., and Galton, D. A.: Histological study of bone marrow regeneration following chemotherapy for acute myeloid leukemia and chronic granulocytic leukemia in blast transformation. Br J Haematol 45:535–540, 1980.
5. Weiss, L.: The hematopoietic microenvironment of the bone marrow. Anat Rec 186:161–184, 1976.

3

LYMPHOPROLIFERATIVE DISEASES

CONCEPT AND SCOPE

The revolution that recast many of the traditional conceptions of lymphoid diseases during the past 25 years can in large part be attributed to the reappraisal of normal and pathological lymph node morphology in the context of new and fundamental observations on lymphocyte physiology and immunology. Many comprehensive reviews and analyses with varying degrees of bias are available on these subjects.[1-3] To the practicing pathologist the contributions of Rappaport have been among the foremost. The acceptance of the nodular and diffuse forms of malignant lymphoid lesions coupled with his emphasis on the cytological characteristics of the participating cells set the stage for most of the practical and meaningful nomenclatures and classifications currently applied to the malignant lymphomas.*[4-8]

The full significance of Rappaport's proposals became evident only when subsequent observations on lymphocyte immunology and transformability were extrapolated to lymphocytic neoplasias. The two major relevant discoveries were that only neoplastic B-lymphocytes gather into more or less discrete aggregates to mimic reactive germinal centers and thereby produce nodular lymphomas and that small lymphocytes, whether B- or T-lymphocytes, can transform into large cells

---

*Rappaport's failure to distinguish the reticulum cell or histiocyte from the subsequently identified transformed lymphocyte must be viewed within the context of the information then available and should not detract from his major contributions.

and thus provide the basis for the cytological variations among the monoclonal lymphocyte proliferations. With respect to the B-lymphocyte the prevailing but as yet unproved view maintains that there is a sequential conversion of the small lymphocyte to the cleaved cell, then to the large cell, and finally to the plasma cell, and that at any point on this continuum a more or less monomorphic clone can develop.[9] In analogy to some carcinoma cells that can mature to produce keratin or form glands, these malignant lymphocytes can also retain some functional properties. Among these are the ability to synthesize immunoglobulins, the capacity to assemble into nodules resembling germinal centers even in extranodal tissues, and the potential to transform to varying degrees to produce either a morphologically homogeneous or a mixed cell population. The T-lymphocyte, though far less commonly a source of lymphomas and leukemias in this country, appears to have a greater functional and immunological complexity than the B-lymphocyte as well as a greater degree of potential cytological heterogeneity.[10] The distinctive morphological features of the neoplastic T-lymphocyte progeny center on the nuclear contour, which may be convoluted, cerebroid, or otherwise contorted. The physiological interaction of the interdigitating and dendritic histiocytes with the T- and B-lymphocytes, respectively, may also be reflected in their lymphomas. This is exemplified by the T cell immunoblastic lymphoma and by some forms of Hodgkin's disease. In both of these conditions morphologically benign histiocytes can be numerous.

A consequence of the monoclonal theory of cancer when applied to hematopoietic malignancies is the consideration of routes of dissemination. Therapeutic decisions are critically influenced by these notions. Generally the route is inferred from study of tumor distribution. For the myeloproliferative diseases this property is relatively obvious, since only the exceptional case originates outside the marrow, and invasion of the blood is the rule. The lymphoproliferative diseases produce a more complex picture. Kaplan has addressed this problem in Hodgkin's disease to develop a rational basis for radiotherapy. He proposes that the disease usually, if not always, originates in a lymph node, most commonly in the cervical or supraclavicular regions, and spreads in a nonrandom pattern to neighboring or distant lymph nodes by way of lymphatic channels.[11] Only when the malignant cells enter the blood via a major lymphatic duct or possibly in the spleen does the disease invade other organs, including the marrow. The low incidence of infiltration into the marrow suggests that blood-stream invasion is an uncommon or a late feature in Hodgkin's disease. Based on similar studies an analogous pattern of sites of origin and routes of dissemination appears to occur in the large cell and poorly differentiated lymphocytic lymphomas. The probability or rapidity of dissemination appears to be greater in poorly differentiated lymphocytic lymphoma than in the large cell lymphoma. By contrast, acute lymphoblastic leukemia and plasma cell myeloma most commonly originate in the marrow, with the lymphoblasts spreading rapidly to all sites through the blood while the plasma cells have a decided propensity to remain confined to the marrow. Chronic lymphocytic leukemia appears to arise with equal ease in the marrow or in a lymph node and accordingly disseminates initially through the blood or lymphatics.

The sequential arrangement of the diseases in this section is rationalized by the lymphoid cell differentiation scheme espoused by Magrath.[12] Differentiation occurs in two successive pathways: (1) the maturation pathway of antigen-independent primary differentiation extending from the as yet unidentified lymphoid stem cell to the immunocompetent but noninscribed well-differentiated lymphocyte of either the B- or T-immunophenotypes and (2) the activation pathway of antigen-dependent secondary differentiation extending beyond the noninscribed well-differen-

tiated lymphocyte either to the inscribed (memory) well-differentiated lymphocyte or to the plasma cell for the B-lymphocyte and to the inscribed well-differentiated lymphocyte for the T-lymphocyte. Extrapolation from this model leads to the conclusion that acute lymphoblastic leukemias and the lymphoblastic lymphomas are diseases derived from cells early in the primary differentiation of the lymphoid cell and that chronic lymphocytic leukemia or well-differentiated lymphocytic lymphoma is a disease of the cell at the final step of this pathway. All other diseases develop from cells in the activation pathway. In hypothetical order they are poorly differentiated lymphocytic lymphoma, large cell lymphoma, and immunoblastic lymphoma followed by either Waldenström's macroglobulinemia or plasma cell myeloma for the B-lymphocyte. For the T-lymphocyte lesions the sequence in the activation pathway is less clear; it includes the cutaneous T cell lymphomas and may terminate with the immunoblastic lymphoma. The cytogenesis of hairy cell leukemia and prolymphocytic leukemia remains unsettled. These conditions may represent aberrations of the noninscribed well-differentiated lymphocyte. Therefore, they follow chronic lymphocytic leukemia in the order of presentation.

Angioimmunoblastic lymphadenopathy is included in this group of diseases because, analogous to the relation of myelodysplasia to myeloblastic leukemia, in some instances it has proved to be a forerunner of immunoblastic lymphoma.

Among the common malignant diseases in the province of the hematologist Hodgkin's disease is the only one whose cell of origin has eluded identification. Currently the major contenders are one form of histiocyte and the T-lymphocyte.[11] Evidence and arguments for each of these cells have been ably presented by their respective proponents. It is ironic that this malignant disease, the first among those of the hematopoietic system to be described, may be the last to find its "parentage." To reflect this state of affairs the section on Hodgkin's disease is placed between those on the lymphoproliferative and the histiocyte proliferative diseases.

The terminology employed to identify each disease does not adhere uncompromisingly to any of several propounded lymphoma classifications.[8] Final selections were based on clarity of communication rather than nosologic purity. An overlay of personal bias is undeniable. When misinterpretation of a designation is possible synonyms are given.

REFERENCES

1. Robb-Smith, A. H. T., and Taylor, C. R.: The classification and nomenclature of the lymphadenopathies. *In* Lymph Node Biopsy. New York, Oxford University Press, 1981, pp. 223–262.
2. Lennert, K.: Histopathology of non-Hodgkin's lymphomas. New York, Springer-Verlag, 1981, pp. 7–21.
3. van den Tweel, J. G., Taylor, C. R., and Bosman, F. T.: Malignant lymphoproliferative diseases. The Hague, Leiden University Press, 1980.
4. Rappaport, H., Winter, W. J., and Hicks, E. B.: Follicular lymphoma: A reevaluation of its position in the scheme of malignant lymphoma based on a survey of 253 cases. Cancer 9:792–821, 1956.
5. Rappaport, H.: Tumors of the hematopoietic system. *In* Atlas of Tumor Pathology. Section 3. Fascicle 8. Washington, D. C., Armed Forces Institute of Pathology, 1966, pp. 1–442.
6. Garvin, A. J., Simon, R., Young, R. C., et al.: The Rappaport classification of non-Hodgkin's lymphomas: A closer look using other proposed classifications. Semin Oncol 7:234–243, 1980.
7. Nathwani, B. N.: A critical analysis of the classifications of non-Hodgkin's lymphomas. Cancer 44:347–384, 1979.
8. The non-Hodgkin's lymphoma pathologic classification project: National Cancer Institute Sponsored Study of Classifications of Non-Hodgkin's Lymphomas. Cancer 49:2112–2135, 1982.
9. Lukes, R. J., and Collins, R. D.: Immunologic characterization of human malignant lymphomas. Cancer 34:1488–1503, 1974.
10. Watanabe, S., Shimosato, Y., and Shimoyama, M.: Lymphoma and leukemia of T-lymphocytes. *In* Sommers, S. C., and Rosen, P. P. (eds.): Pathology Annual. Vol. 16. Part 2. New York, Appleton-Century-Crofts, 1981, pp. 155–203.
11. Kaplan, H. S.: Hodgkin's Disease. Cambridge, Harvard University Press, 1980.
12. Magrath, I. T.: Lymphocyte differentiation: An essential basis for the comprehension of lymphoid neoplasia. J Natl Cancer Inst 67:501–514, 1981.

ACUTE LYMPHOBLASTIC LEUKEMIA

The morphological simplicity of the leukemic cells in this disease belies their immunological and chemical diversity. As the hypothetical pleuripotential stem cell, as yet cytologically elusive, matures to the recognizable lymphoblast, it gains and loses antigenic and enzymatic markers. A bewildering array of potential leukemic phenotypes is thereby created.[1] To date, the immunological classification comprising four subgroups—common acute lymphoblastic leukemia (common-ALL), T-ALL, B-ALL, and unclassifiable-ALL—appears to be the most useful therapeutically. These subgroups represent approximately 70, 15, 5, and 10 per cent, respectively, of cases over the entire age range.[2, 3] The disease, however, is most prevalent in infants and children. Cytologically three subgroups are recognized by the French-American-British classification scheme—L-1, the homogeneous, small lymphoblastic; L-2, the heterogeneous, large lymphoblastic; and L-3, the Burkitt type.[4, 5] There appears to be only limited correlation between cell morphology and immunological phenotype.[2]

The value of the core marrow biopsy in this disease is not different from that of leukemia in general; namely, it is useful for both diagnosis and therapeutic monitoring. For anatomical reasons, however, core biopsy is not generally done for diagnostic purposes in patients younger than 15 years unless aspiration is fruitless. The "dry tap" is due either to marked hypocellularity[6] or to packing of the cells into an unyielding fibrillar meshwork of a very hypercellular marrow.[7] In pediatric patients most biopsies are done to determine the possibility of relapse rather than the presence of remission.

In the core specimen the marrow is almost invariably hypercellular with the intertrabecular space usually being totally filled and the leukemic cells almost always being the sole occupants. Corresponding to the FAB classification there are three subgroups. The *first group* is readily recognized by the striking monotony and homogeneity of the leukemic cells. The characteristic cell is of intermediate size, falling between the size of the well-differentiated lymphocyte and the large transformed lymphocyte, and is essentially filled by a round nucleus having a thin nuclear membrane and containing dispersed chromatin but no visible nucleolus (Figs. 3–1A and B). This corresponds to the L-1 type in the FAB classification. The *second group* is characterized by its heterogeneity on the basis of variation of nuclear size and shape. The cells and their nuclei are generally larger than those of the first group, with nuclear dents and folds being conspicuous. Cytoplasm and nucleoli are also more obvious in contrast to the first group (Figs. 3–2A and B). This group corresponds to the L-2 type. These cases can be easily confused with those of acute myeloblastic leukemia in which no maturation is present. Cytochemical and immunological phenotyping techniques applied to aspirated cells may be necessary for a

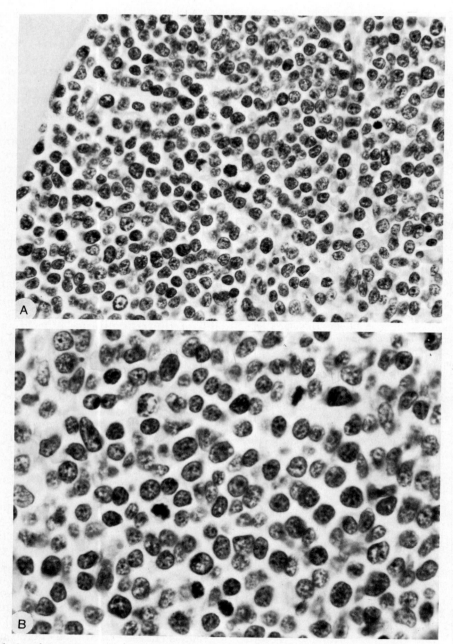

Figure 3–1. *A* and *B*. Designated as L-1 in the FAB classification, this form of acute lymphoblastic leukemia has a remarkably uniform cell population. The discrete round nuclei have a cross-sectional area approximately 50 per cent greater than the well-differentiated lymphocyte's and are filled with finely textured, uniformly distributed chromatin. Little, if any, cytoplasm is evident. Mitoses are frequent. 680×, 1000×, hematoxylin and eosin stain (H&E).

reliable diagnosis. The *third group* is *Burkitt's lymphoma,* in which the marrow morphology is identical to that of the more common extramedullary disease except for the absence of the tingible histiocytes. The L-3 lymphoblast simulates the L-1 type, but its nuclear chromatin is more particulate, and its nucleoli are obvious (Figs. 3–3*A* and *B*).

Cytoplasmic vacuoles cannot be discerned, as a rule, in the core section.

The best established correlations between morphology and immunology exist for Burkitt's lymphoma cells that are B-lymphoblasts[8] and for cells with convoluted nuclei that are T-lymphoblasts.[8] The latter, however, can also have round nuclei. Lymphoblasts with

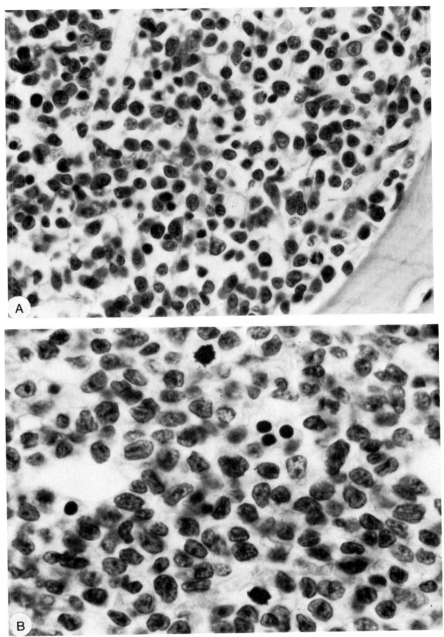

Figure 3–2. *A* and *B*. This form is known as L-2 in the FAB classification. Its cells have somewhat irregularly shaped nuclei whose chromatin is slightly coarser than that of the L-1 cell. In some cells a nucleolus is evident. Some of these nucleolated cells are indistinguishable from and may be prolymphocytes. Cytoplasm is also more obvious in this form than in the L-1 type. Mitoses are frequent. 680×, 1000×, H&E.

the common antigen can belong to either the first or second group of the FAB scheme.[2]

Lymphoblastic lymphoma is most probably a clinically rather than a biologically distinctive disease differing from acute lymphoblastic leukemia only in mode of presentation. Lymphoblastic lymphoma most commonly appears as enlarged supradiaphragmatic lymph nodes or as a mediastinal or abdominal tumor. This difference can be viewed as analogous to the relation between chronic lymphocytic leukemia and well-differentiated lymphocytic lymphoma.

Differential diagnostic considerations are age related. In infants and children the diseases that may involve the marrow and mimic

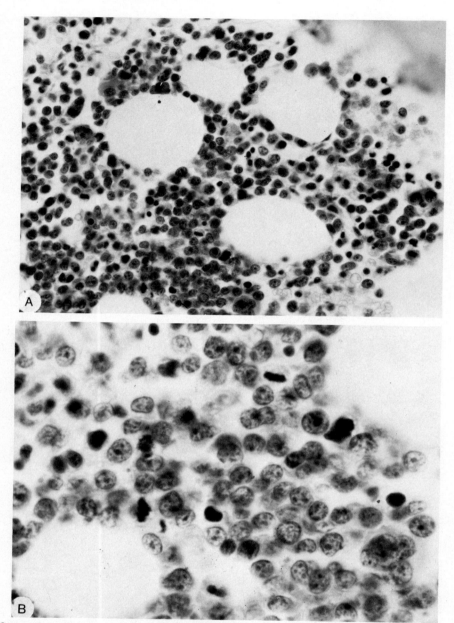

Figure 3–3. *A* and *B*. The Burkitt's form of acute lymphoblast leukemia is known as L-3 in the FAB system. The cells closely simulate the L-1 lymphoblast in size, shape, and uniformity of nuclei. In the Burkitt's cell, however, the chromatin is more particulate than dusty in texture, and small nucleoli are obvious. Vacuolation of the cytoplasm is not easily visualized in the core biopsy sections. Mitoses are frequent. 680×, 1000×, H&E.

acute lymphoblastic leukemia are neuroblastoma, Ewing's tumor, rhabdomyoblastoma, and medulloblastoma. In adults the small cell undifferentiated carcinoma of the lung may do likewise. The immunoperoxidase technique for the demonstration of terminal deoxynucleotidyl transferase, present in the majority of cases of acute lymphoblastic leukemia, can be useful in distinguishing this disease from the metastatic cancers as well as from acute myeloblastic leukemia.[9, 10]

REFERENCES

1. Magrath, I. T.: Lymphocyte differentiation: An essential basis for the comprehension of lymphoid neoplasia. J Natl Canc Inst 67:501–514, 1981.
2. Greaves, M. F., Janossy, G., Peto, J., et al.: Immunologically defined subclasses of acute lympho-

blastic leukemia in children. Br J Haematol 48:179–197, 1981.

3. Willemze, R.: The prognostic relevance of leukemic cell typing in acute lymphoblastic leukemia. *In* van den Tweel, J. G., Taylor, C. R., and Bosman, F. T. (eds.): Malignant Lymphoproliferative Diseases. The Hague, Leiden University Press, 1980, pp. 481–487.

4. Bennett, J. M., Catovsky, D., Daniel, M. T., et al.: Proposals for the classification of the acute leukemias. Br J Haematol 33:451–458, 1976.

5. Gralnick, H. R., Galton, D. A. G., Catovsky, D., et al.: Classification of acute leukemia. Ann Intern Med 87:740–753, 1977.

6. Breatnach, F., Chessells, J. M., and Greaves, M. F.: The aplastic presentation of childhood leukemia: A feature of common-ALL. Br J Haematol 49:387–393, 1981.

7. Hann, I. M., Evan, D. I. K., Marsden, H. B., et al.: Bone marrow fibrosis in acute lymphoblastic leukaemia of childhood. J Clin Pathol 31:313–315, 1978.

8. Williams, A. H., Taylor, G. R., Higgins, G. R., et al.: Childhood lymphoma-leukemia. Cancer 42:171–181, 1978.

9. Stass, S. A., Dean, L., Peiper, S. C., et al.: Determination of terminal deoxynucleotidyl transferase on bone marrow smears by immunoperoxidase. Am J Clin Pathol 77:174–176, 1982.

10. Halverson, C. A., Falini, B., Taylor, C. R., et al.: Detection of terminal transferase in paraffin sections with the immunoperoxidase technique. Am J Pathol 105:241–254, 1981.

LYMPHOBLASTIC LYMPHOMA

The several extant classifications of lymphomas have fruitfully produced a large number of names for a numerically small group of lesions that could probably be better designated as lymphoblastic lymphoma followed by an appropriate qualifier.[1, 2] Among the names assigned to these lesions are lymphoblastic lymphoma, convoluted and nonconvoluted types; convoluted T cell lymphoma; undifferentiated lymphoma, Burkitt's and non-Burkitt's types; small noncleaved follicular center cell lymphoma; and lymphoblastic lymphoma, Burkitt's and other B cell types. Clinical, morphological, and immunological data can be mustered to support the proposal that these lymphomas are either closely related to or actually represent subgroups of the far more common disease, acute lymphoblastic leukemia.[3] The therapeutically and prognostically useful subgrouping of the latter disease by cytological and immunological features is generally recognized. Subgrouping may also prove cogent in the lymphoblastic lymphomas.

In this group of lymphomas a mediastinal or abdominal mass without initial involvement of the peripheral blood and marrow is a conspicuous clinical finding, a high mitotic index with blastic cells a conspicuous histological finding, and a differentiation along the B- or T-lymphocyte pathway an almost constant immunological finding.

Four morphologically recognized lymphomas are included in this group. The first type is known as the *convoluted cell form* (Fig. 3–4).[4–7] Clinically, the presence of a mediastinal mass or lymph node enlargement, or both, in the absence of leukemic peripheral blood is most characteristic. Almost consistently, however, the marrow soon becomes filled with lymphoblasts, and a leukemic phase supervenes. The prevailing cell, the convoluted lymphoblast, has an irregular lobulated nucleus of intermediate size with creases and folds and finely dispersed chromatin and lacks distinct nucleoli. Cytoplasm is scanty, and cell borders are not visible. Mitoses are abundant. Evidence obtained from pediatric and adult cases indicates that this lesion arises predominantly from the T-lymphocyte.

The second type, the *nonconvoluted* or *round cell form,* is clinically indistinguishable from the convoluted cell form (Fig. 3–5).[4, 7] The principal cell is characterized by a round nucleus of intermediate size that contains dispersed chromatin and is surrounded by virtually no visible cytoplasm. Nucleoli may or may not be visible. Mitoses are abundant. In the marrow core specimen this round lymphoblast cannot be cytologically distinguished from the cell of the more frequently occurring acute lymphoblastic leukemia without the mediastinal mass or lymph node enlargement. Immunologically this subgroup appears to be more heterogeneous than the preceding one and to include pre-B, B, T, and non-B non-T phenotypes.

The third type is generally known as *Burkitt's lymphoma* (Fig. 3–6).[7–10] Clinically, the disease in this country is commonly manifested by an abdominal tumor usually produced by an intestinal or ovarian lesion. Unlike the other lymphomas in this group, Burkitt's lymphoma is almost exclusively limited to children and young adults. The marrow is involved initially in about 20 per cent of cases, and in some of these the cells appear in the peripheral blood, albeit infrequently in leukemic proportions. There is universal agreement that this is a B cell lymphoma with immunoglobulin production and the presence of specific surface antigens being char-

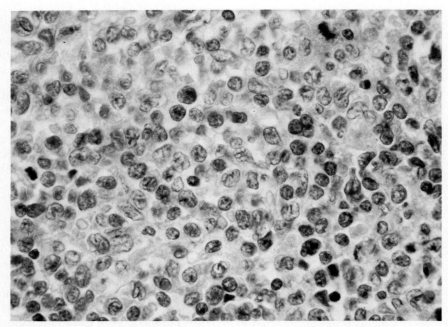

Figure 3–4. Lymphoblastic lymphoma of the convoluted cell type. The deep narrow grooves produce the characteristic convoluted shape in the nucleus, whose size is intermediate between that of the well-differentiated and the large noncleaved lymphocyte. Nuclear chromatin is particulate and dispersed, and nucleoli are barely, if at all, visible. Mitoses are common. 680×, H&E.

acteristic of the causative cell. In view of these functions the designation of the cell in the antigenically common acute lymphoblastic leukemia as a lymphoblast and the cell in Burkitt's lymphomas as undifferentiated is inconsistent and misleading. By analogy, the carcinoma is designated as undifferentiated only when no evidence of function such as gland formation or mucin or keratin production is detected. The FAB classification of acute leukemia recognizes the cell in Burkitt's lymphoma as a lymphoblast, and some lym-

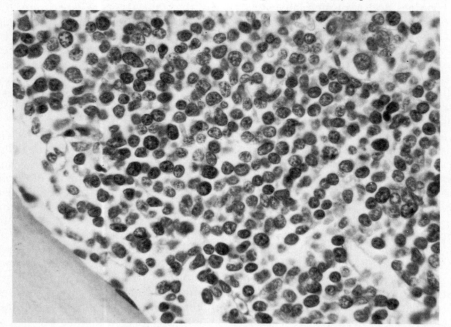

Figure 3–5. Lymphoblastic lymphoma of the nonconvoluted or round cell type. See the discussion of lymphoblastic leukemia, L-1 type. 680×, H&E.

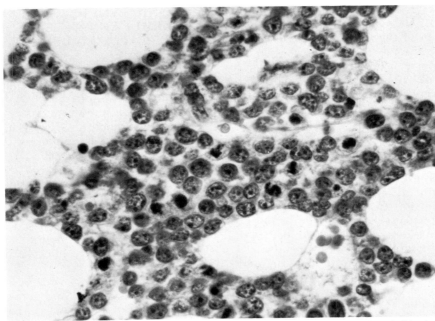

Figure 3–6. Lymphoblastic lymphoma of the Burkitt's type. See the discussion of acute lymphoblastic leukemia, L-3 type. 1000×, H&E.

phoma classifications also designate the lesion as a lymphoblastic lymphoma.

The fourth and final type is the *pleomorphic form* (Fig. 3–7).[7–11] The argument of differentiation also attests to the current inadequacy of the designation, undifferentiated lymphoma, non-Burkitt's type, for this lesion. The disease is not as homogeneous morphologically or immunologically as Burkitt's lymphoma, but production of surface antigen or immunoglobulin is documented. Like Burkitt's lymphoma this disease commonly

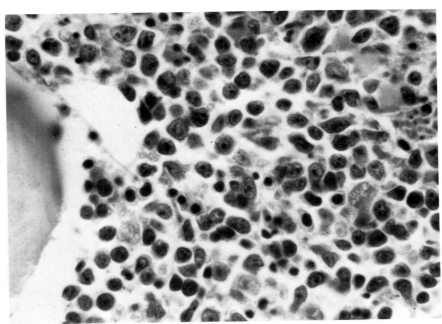

Figure 3–7. Lymphoblastic lymphoma of the pleomorphic type. The variation in nuclear sizes and shapes when compared with the two lesions shown in Figures 3–5 and 3–6 is obvious. Nucleolar and chromatin detail, however, mimic that of the Burkitt's lymphoma but differ remarkably from that of the round cell type. 680×, H&E.

appears as an abdominal mass, but unlike Burkitt's lymphoma it has no age specificity. Involvement of the marrow is the least common in this disease group, occurring in only about 15 per cent of cases. Morphologically in the marrow the lesion has both similarities and differences with respect to the other lymphomas in this group. The cell nuclei are approximately the same size as those of Burkitt's disease, but in contrast to the monomorphism of the Burkitt's and round cell forms, that is, the L-3 and L-1 lymphoblasts, respectively, the cells are pleomorphic in cell and nuclear size and shape. On the other hand, distinction from the L-2 lymphoblast can be problematic. Undoubtedly, some cases that involve the marrow are identified as the L-2 type of lymphoblastic leukemia.

The differential diagnostic considerations in evaluating the marrow core specimen are the same as those given for acute lymphoblastic leukemia.

REFERENCES

1. Nathwani, B. N.: A critical analysis of the classifications of non-Hodgkin's lymphomas. Cancer 44:347–384, 1979.
2. The non-Hodgkin's lymphoma pathologic classification project: National Cancer Institute Sponsored Study of Classifications of Non-Hodgkin's Lymphomas. Cancer 49:2112–2135, 1982.
3. Magrath, I. T.: Lymphocyte differentiation: An essential basis for the comprehension of lymphoid neoplasia. J Natl Canc Inst 67:501–514, 1981.
4. Nathwani, B. N., Kim, H., and Rappaport, H.: Malignant lymphoma, lymphoblastic. Cancer 38:964–983, 1976.
5. Williams, A. H., Taylor, C. R., Higgins, G. R., et al.: Childhood lymphoma-leukemia. Cancer 42:171–181, 1978.
6. Rosen, P. J., Feinstein, D. I., Pattengale, P. K., et al.: Convoluted lymphocytic lymphoma in adults. Ann Intern Med 89:319–324, 1978.
7. Kjeldsberg, C. R., Wilson, J. F., and Berard, C. W.: Non-Hodgkin's lymphoma in children. Hum Pathol 14:612–627, 1983.
8. Arseneau, J. C., Canellos, G. P., Banks, P. M., et al.: American Burkitt's lymphoma: A clinicopathologic study of 30 cases. 1. Am J Med 58:314–321, 1975.
9. Banks, P. M., Arseneau, J. C., Gralnick, H. R., et al.: American Burkitt's lymphoma: A clinicopathologic study of 30 cases. 2. Am J Med 58:322–329, 1975.
10. Miliauskas, J. R., Berard, C. W., Young, R. C., et al.: Undifferentiated non-Hodgkin's lymphomas (Burkitt's and non-Burkitt's types). Cancer 50:2115–2121, 1982.
11. Grogan, T. M., Warnke, R. A., and Kaplan, H. S.: A comparative study of Burkitt's and non-Burkitt's "undifferentiated" malignant lymphoma. Cancer 49:1817–1828, 1982.

CHRONIC LYMPHOCYTIC LEUKEMIA AND WELL-DIFFERENTIATED LYMPHOCYTIC LYMPHOMA

Chronic lymphocytic leukemia and well-differentiated lymphocytic lymphoma represent neoplastic proliferations of cells recognized morphologically as well differentiated, small, or mature lymphocytes. Although by tradition these lymphocytes are considered mature, according to current immunological views they are immature and fail to undergo immunological maturation when appropriately stimulated. By convention, chronic lymphocytic leukemia is diagnosed on the basis of features of the peripheral blood, whereas well-differentiated lymphocytic lymphoma is diagnosed from typical lymph node histopathology. Prevailing concepts view these manifestations as the fluid and solid phases, respectively, of one disease that may have several sequential patterns of evolution and that in some cases ultimately show the disease in both the leukemic and lymphomatous forms.[1]

The B-lymphocyte is the source of the neoplastic clone in the great majority of cases. Only the exceptional case in this country stems from the T-lymphocyte—an observation differing remarkably from findings in Japan. The most common sites of development of the monoclone appear to be a lymph node or the marrow. Estimates from published data indicate that the former occurs with a minimal frequency of about 25 per cent[2] and the latter, 15 to 20 per cent.[3] In the remainder and probably the majority of cases both of these sites are afflicted at the time of initial diagnosis whether or not the disease is evident in the peripheral blood. The leukemic phase rarely occurs without marrow involvement even in the presence of nodal disease.[2] Conversely, only about half of the cases with marrow infiltration display leukemia.[4]

In ascertaining marrow involvement in the lymphoproliferative diseases studies have established the superior efficiency of the core biopsy over aspiration, whether the aspirated particles are studied by smear or section.[5] Smears can be especially misleading because a single marrow particle containing a lymphocyte aggregate can be misinterpreted as representative of the entire marrow.

A classification scheme of marrow involvement based on the intensity and pattern of marrow infiltration has been proposed by Rywlin[6] and with minor modifications applied by several investigators to core biopsy specimens.[3, 7, 8] Four patterns of involvement may be recognized:

1. Interstitial. Lymphocytes permeate the stroma between the fat cells with a proportionate loss of normal hematopoietic cells but with limited loss of fat cells (Fig. 3–8A). In practice, at least 30 per cent of the hematopoietic cells should be lymphocytes before neoplastic involvement can be diagnosed with almost complete assurance.

2. Nodular. Densely packed aggregates of lymphocytes punctuate the marrow with a limited loss of fat cells (Fig. 3–8B). A minimum of five nodules should be present in a single core specimen in order that marrow involvement be diagnosed.

3. Mixed. A combination of interstitial and nodular forms is associated with a moderate loss of hematopoietic and fat cells.

4. Diffuse. Interstitial or nodular, or both, forms are present with virtual or complete filling of the marrow space by lymphocytes (Fig. 3–8C). The term "nodular" in this context is unrelated to and is not to be confused with its meaning or significance in the lymph node pathology of lymphomas. "Focal" or "multifocal" would be a less ambiguous term. Correlation studies have shown that the interstitial and nodular patterns tend to occur when clinically evident disease is limited and that the diffuse pattern is usually present in the advanced stages.[3, 7, 8] Even more important, however, is the proportion of lymphocytes relative to the remaining hematopoietic cells irrespective of the pattern. Deleterious cytopenias of the myeloid lineages can develop in the peripheral blood in the limited as well as the diffuse patterns if the myeloid precursors have been substantially replaced by the lymphocytes or by fat cells. This feature is critical in distinguishing replacement cytopenias from immune cytopenias, which can also complicate this disease. The latter type may be reflected by a hyperplasia of the relevant precursors (Fig. 3–9). There is no correlation between the pattern or intensity of marrow infiltration and the presentation of the disease as a leukemia or a lymphoma.

Cytological uniformity is the rule in the interstitial pattern or the interstitial component of the mixed pattern in which the well-differentiated lymphocytes crowd between the fat cells (Fig. 3–10). By contrast, the nodules commonly contain central areas composed of larger and slightly pleomorphic cells with vesicular nuclei with or without nucleoli (Figs. 3–11A and B). Analogous foci in lymph nodes of well-differentiated lymphoma have been designated as pseudofollicular proliferation or growth centers.

In rare cases of this disease the lymphocytes in the marrow and blood contain cytoplasmic amorphous or crystalline inclusions of immunoglobulin (Ig) (Fig. 3–12).[9–11] This has proved in most instances to be either IgM λ, IgM κ, or IgA λ. This feature serves as evidence for the B cell nature of the monoclone and its kinship to the plasma cell and also demonstrates a defect related to dissociation of protein synthesis from protein secretion in these cells. Similar inclusions have been reported in Waldenström's macroglobulinemia and are more widely known for their occurrence in the plasma cells.

Evolution to large cell lymphoma is a classic, albeit uncommon, terminating phase of chronic lymphocytic leukemia (Figs. 3–13A and B).[12, 13] This sequence is known as Richter's syndrome. Even more unusual is the more recently described prolymphocytic evolution[14] and progression to blast cell crisis.[15]

The problem of distinguishing the normal lymphocyte content of the marrow from the state designated as lymphoid hyperplasia and the latter from neoplasia has been addressed by several investigators.[6, 16] The normal hematopoietic cell population includes from 10 to 16 per cent lymphocytes. These may be dispersed or in the form of small aggregates. The latter type has been identified in almost 50 per cent of an adult hospital population selected for marrow examination but having no evidence of lymphoma or leukemia. Characteristically the aggregates are small, clearly delineated, show no tendency to spread between adjacent fat cells, and occur with a frequency of 1 to 3 per core specimen (Fig. 3–14). Rarely are reaction centers present (Fig. 3–15). The presence of somewhat greater numbers of lymphocytes has been considered to indicate hyperplasia, but the distinction between the normal state and hyperplasia is arbitrary, as is the border between hyperplasia and neoplasia. Hyperplasia is most frequently associated with rheumatoid arthritis, hyperthyroidism, and hemolytic anemia. Attempts to discriminate objectively between the normal or hyperplastic lymphocyte content and leukemic or lymphomatous involvement have utilized immu-

Text continued on page 67

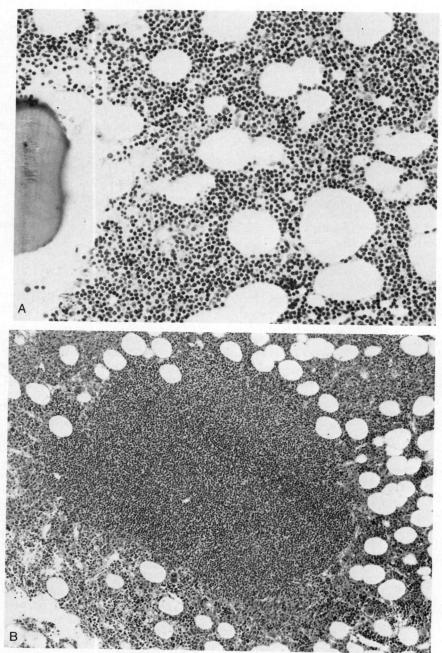

Figure 3–8. *A, B,* and *C.* Interstitial, focal, and diffuse patterns of distribution in the marrow of chronic lymphocytic leukemia or well-differentiated lymphocytic lymphoma. 250×, 100× and 100×, H&E.

Illustration continued on opposite page

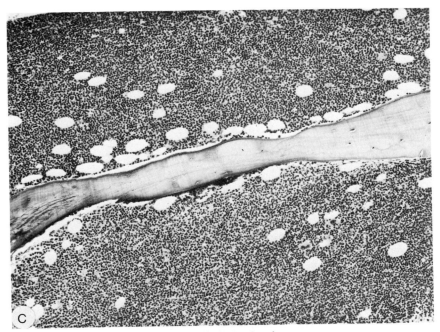

Figure 3–8. *Continued.*

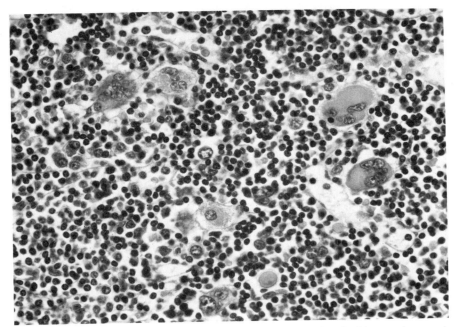

Figure 3–9. Diffuse involvement by chronic lymphocytic leukemia associated with megakaryocytic hyperplasia related to hypersplenic sequestration of platelets, immune destruction, or both. 400×, H&E.

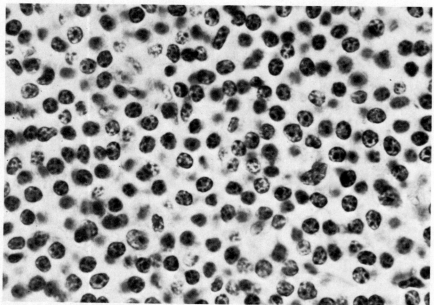

Figure 3–10. Coarse blocks of chromatin in uniformly round nuclei that lack nucleoli and show no mitotic activity are characteristic of well-differentiated lymphocytes. 1000×, H&E.

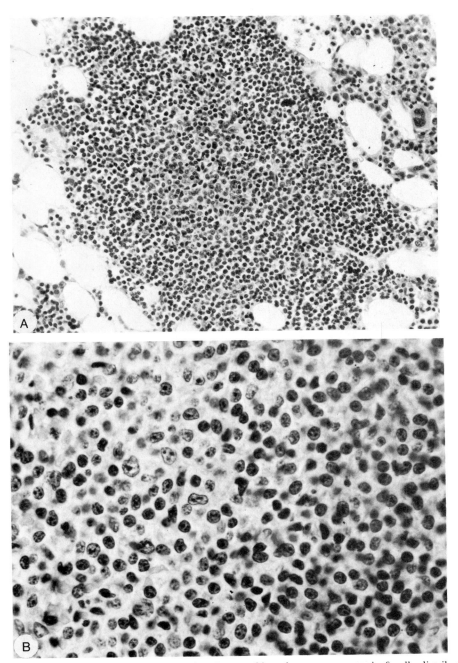

Figure 3–11. *A* and *B*. Growth center and peripheral zone of lymphocyte aggregate in focally distributed chronic lymphocytic leukemia. The peripheral zone is populated by well-differentiated lymphocytes, whereas the growth center includes larger lymphocytes having vesicular nuclei containing nucleoli. Individually, some of the latter are indistinguishable from prolymphocytes and large transformed lymphocytes. No mitoses are present. 250× and 680×, H&E.

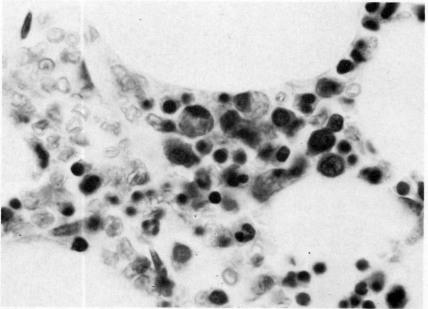

Figure 3–12. Crystals of IgM κ fill the cytoplasm and displace the nucleus to the cell margin in a case of chronic lymphocytic leukemia. 1000×, H&E.

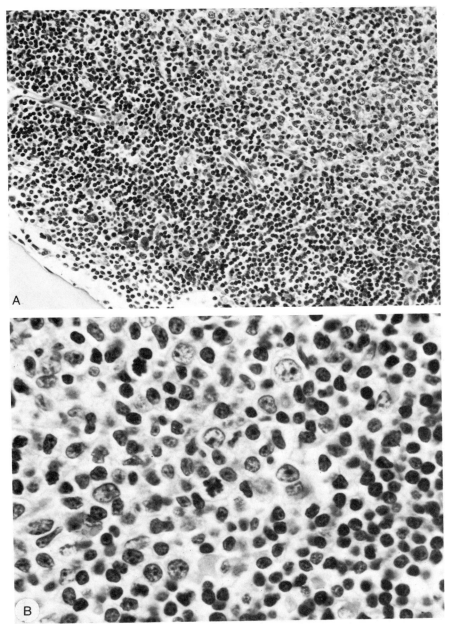

Figure 3–13. *A* and *B*. Chronic lymphocytic leukemia progressing to large cell lymphoma (Richter's syndrome) is indicated by extensive areas of well-differentiated lymphocytes heavily admixed with or replaced by small cleaved and large lymphocytes adjacent to areas consisting of only well-differentiated lymphocytes. Cells in mitosis are present only in the areas of progression. 250× and 800×, H&E.

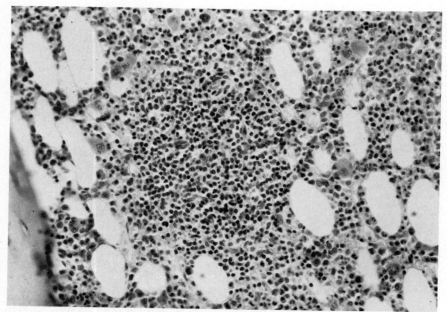

Figure 3–14. A small aggregate of well-differentiated lymphocytes in the otherwise unremarkable marrow sample from a patient with chronic rheumatoid arthritis. 250×, H&E.

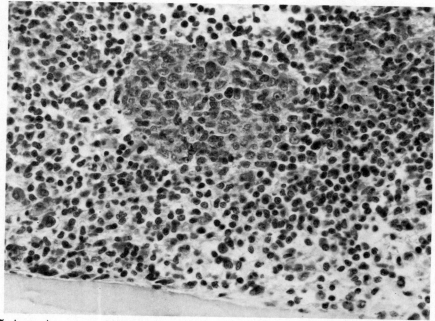

Figure 3–15. A reaction center within an aggregate of well-differentiated lymphocytes in the marrow of an elderly patient with chronic rheumatoid arthritis. 400×, H&E.

nocytological procedures.[17, 18] This has been done using formalin-fixed[17] and frozen[18] marrow tissue. Unfortunately, the formalin-fixed tissue is limited to the detection of cytoplasmic immunoglobulin, whereas the frozen tissue, by which the more pertinent surface immunoglobulin can be demonstrated, involves a laborious and time-consuming preparation.

REFERENCES

1. Rundles, R. W.: Chronic lymphocytic leukemia. *In* Williams, W. J., Beutler, E., Erslev, A. J., and Lichtman, M. A. (eds.): Hematology. New York, McGraw-Hill, 1983, pp. 981–998.
2. Pangalis, G. A., Nathwani, B. N., and Rappaport, H.: Malignant lymphoma, well differentiated lymphocytic. Cancer 39:999–1010, 1977.
3. Lipshutz, M. D., Rabia, M., Rai, K. R., et al.: Bone marrow biopsy and clinical staging in chronic lymphocytic leukemia. Cancer 46:1422–1427, 1980.
4. Foucar, K., McKenna, R. W., Frizzera, G., et al.: Incidence and patterns of bone marrow and blood involvement by lymphoma in relationship to the Lukes-Collins classification. Blood 54:1417–1422, 1979.
5. Coller, B. S., Chabner, B. A., and Gralnick, H. R.: Frequencies and patterns of bone marrow involvement in non-Hodgkin lymphoma. Am J Hematol 3:105–119, 1977.
6. Rywlin, A. M.: Histopathology of the bone marrow. Boston, Little, Brown & Company, 1976, pp. 95–113.
7. Rozman, C., Hernandez-Nieto, L., Monserrat, E., et al.: Prognostic significance of bone marrow patterns in chronic lymphocytic leukaemia. Br J Haematol 47:529–537, 1981.
8. Bartl, R., Frisch, B., Burkhardt, R., et al.: Assessment of marrow trephine in relation to staging in chronic lymphocytic leukaemia. Br J Haematol 51:1–15, 1982.
9. Clark, C., Rydell, R. E., Kaplan, M. E.: Frequent association of IgM λ with crystalline inclusions in chronic lymphatic leukemia lymphocytes. N Engl J Med 289:113–117, 1973.
10. Gordon, J., and Smith, J. L.: Characterization of a secretory block in a case of CLL with IgA λ crystalline inclusions. Br J Haematol 43:155–158, 1979.
11. Nies, K. M., Marshall, J., Oberlin, A., et al.: Chronic lymphocytic leukemia with gamma chain cytoplasmic inclusions. Am J Clin Pathol 65:948–956, 1976.
12. Nowell, P., Finan, J., Glover, D., et al.: Cytogenetic evidence for the clonal nature of Richter's syndrome. Blood 58:183–186, 1981.
13. Harousseau, J. L., Flandrin, G., Tricot, G., et al.: Malignant lymphoma supervening in chronic lymphocytic leukemia and related disorders. Cancer 48:1302–1308, 1981.
14. Enno, A., Catovsky, D., O'Brien, M., et al.: "Prolymphocytoid" transformation of chronic lymphocytic leukaemia. Br J Haematol 41:9–18, 1979.
15. Brouet, J. C., Preud'Homme, J. L., Seligmann, M., et al.: Blast cells with monoclonal surface immunoglobulin in two cases of acute blast crisis supervening on chronic lymphocytic leukaemia. Br Med J 4:23–24, 1973.
16. Maeda, K., Hyun, B. H., and Rebuck, J. W.: Lymphoid follicles in bone marrow aspirates. Am J Clin Pathol 67:41–48, 1977.
17. Hitzman, J., Li, C. Y., and Kyle, R.: Immunoperoxidase staining of bone marrow sections. Cancer 48:2438–2446, 1981.
18. Pizzolo, G., Chilosi, M., Cetto, G. L., et al.: Immunohistological analysis of bone marrow involvement in lympho-proliferative disorders. Br J Haematol 50:95–100, 1982.

PROLYMPHOCYTIC LEUKEMIA

This uncommon form of leukemia was distinguished from simulating types of lymphoid leukemias relatively recently.[1] The basis for its acceptance as an entity rests not only on special clinical and laboratory features but also on failure to respond to conventional chemotherapy.[1, 2] Characteristically the disease occurs during or beyond the fourth decade of life and is manifested by moderate to marked splenomegaly, little or no lymph node enlargement, and marked and persistent blood lymphocytosis. The morphology of the prolymphocyte is the keystone of the diagnosis. It has been succinctly described and clearly demonstrated to be different from the well-differentiated lymphocyte, the lymphoblast, the lymphosarcoma cell, and the hairy cell. Immunologically the monoclonal proliferation may be of the B or T type of lymphoid cell, and in the latter type both helper and suppressor varieties have been recorded.[3]

Evolution from chronic lymphocytic leukemia to prolymphocytic leukemia has been described.[4] This may be viewed as analogous to the more commonly occurring blast cell crisis of chronic granulocytic leukemia.

The marrow is invariably affected. It is laden with varying numbers of prolymphocytes distributed in a diffuse or focal fashion. Recognition of the prolymphocyte in the marrow core section is based on its distinctive nucleus, which is intermediate in size between the well-differentiated and the large noncleaved lymphocytes and round to oval in shape and has a conspicuous albeit small nucleolus, a small amount of particulate chromatin, and a distinct nuclear membrane (Figs. 3–16*A*, *B*, and *C*). An incomplete cytoplasmic rim may be evident. The number of mitoses is increased but less so than in acute lymphoblastic leukemia or lymphoblas-

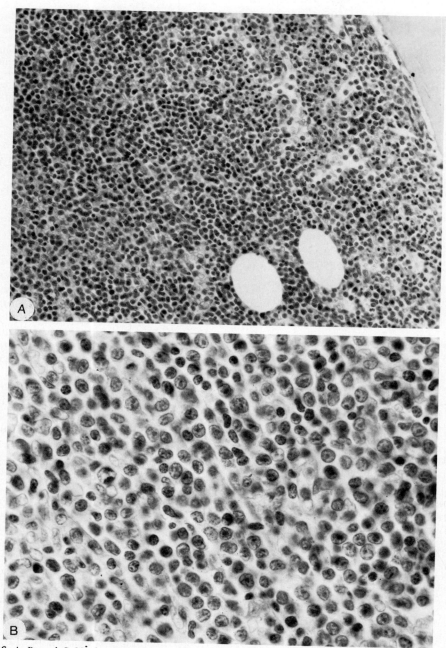

Figure 3–16. *A, B,* and *C.* Nuclear characteristics are most important in distinguishing the prolymphocyte from its lymphoid colleagues. These features include size, which is between that of the well-differentiated and of the large noncleaved lymphocyte, shape, which is round to oval, chromatin, which is sparse and particulate, and a nucleolus, which is small but conspicuous. 250×, 680×, and 1000×, H&E.

Illustration continued on opposite page

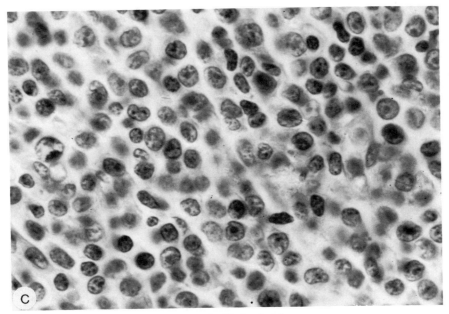

Figure 3–16. *Continued.*

tic lymphoma. A minor admixture of the prolymphocyte population with well-differentiated lymphocytes, small and large cleaved lymphocytes, or large noncleaved lymphocytes serves to emphasize the idiotypicality of the prolymphocyte and to facilitate its recognition.

In differential diagnosis this leukemia is most readily confused with chronic lymphocytic leukemia or the diffusely infiltrating form of poorly differentiated lymphocytic lymphoma. The distinction from lymphoblastic lymphoma or leukemia is more obvious. Careful attention to nuclear size and shape, chromatin density, and presence of nucleoli is necessary. Confirmation of the diagnosis by study of a smear preparation of blood or marrow may be required.

REFERENCES

1. Galton, D. A. G., Goldman, J. M., Wiltshaw, E., et al.: Prolymphocytic leukaemia. Br J Haematol 27:7–23, 1974.
2. Bearman, R. M., Pangalis, G. A., and Rappaport, H.: Prolymphocytic leukemia. Cancer 42:2360–2372, 1978.
3. Chan, W. C., Check, I. J., Heffner, L. T., et al.: Prolymphocytic leukemia of helper cell phenotype. Am J Clin Pathol 77:643–647, 1982.
4. Enno, A., Catovsky, D., O'Brien, M., et al.: "Prolymphocytoid" transformation of chronic lymphocytic leukaemia. Br J Haematol 41:9–18, 1979.

HAIRY CELL LEUKEMIA

A provisional diagnosis of hairy cell leukemia based on the presence of splenomegaly and pancytopenia with abnormal leukocytes in the peripheral blood should be substantiated by the presence of characteristic pathology in a marrow core specimen.[1-4] Although the monocyte has been implicated, the B-lymphocyte is currently the acknowledged causative cell in most cases and the T-lymphocyte rarely so.[5] Marrow involvement can be expected in all cases. Since aspiration of the marrow is futile as a rule, the core biopsy is a definitive diagnostic procedure.

All descriptions of the histopathology are in essential agreement.[2, 3] The marrow is focally or extensively occupied by bland-appearing mononuclear cells embedded in a network of fine fibrils (Figs. 3–17 and 3–18). Characteristically the cell nuclei are round to oval or slightly indented and irregular and appear as if surrounded by a clear or pale cytoplasmic halo. Nuclear chromatin is finely stippled, nucleoli are indistinct if present, and mitoses are rare. The cell borders cannot be optically resolved from the fibrillar net-

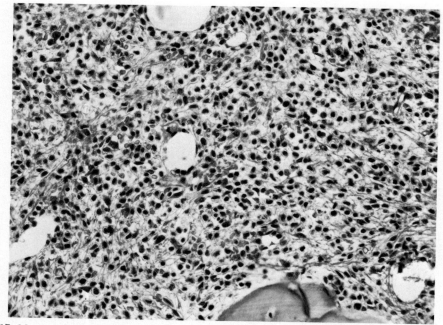

Figure 3–17. Mononuclear relatively uniform cells are distributed with considerable regularity in a fine fibrillar network. All normal hematopoietic cells and most fat cells have been replaced. 250×, H&E.

work, and the hairy processes that typify the malignant cells in the peripheral blood are not demonstrable in the standard histological sections examined by light microscopy. The reticulin stain reveals a loosely woven net of fine fibrils that appear to envelop almost each individual cell. There is no collagen fibrosis.

In the differential diagnostic considerations distinction of hairy cell leukemia from well-differentiated, poorly differentiated, or

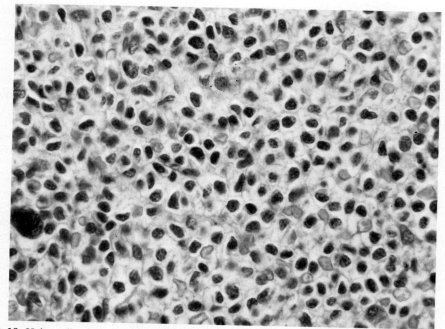

Figure 3–18. Hairy cells possess single round to oval and sometimes angulated nuclei surrounded by an optically clear cytoplasmic space that is delineated by the fibrillar network of reticulin. Nucleoli are not evident. Mitoses are rarely present. There is no collagen. 680×, H&E.

large cell (histiocytic) lymphoma or acute lymphoblastic leukemia is rarely difficult.[3, 4] The well-differentiated lymphocyte is smaller and has a more uniformly round nucleus with denser, more darkly staining chromatin. In poorly differentiated lymphocytic lymphoma clusters of the malignant cells are usually paratrabecular in location, and the cells are smaller and their nuclei smaller, more irregular, and angulated. The large cell lymphoma has cells with either large rounded vesicular nuclei containing conspicuous nucleoli or large cleaved nuclei. The latter may simulate hairy cells but lack the enmeshing fibrillar net and cytoplasmic space. Finally, aside from obvious cytological differences, a high mitotic index readily distinguishes the lymphoblastic lymphomas and leukemias from hairy cell leukemia.

REFERENCES

1. Golomb, H. M.: Hairy Cell Leukemia. *In* Williams, W. J., Beulter, E., Erslev, A. J., and Lichtman, M. A. (eds.): Hematology. New York, McGraw-Hill, 1983, pp. 999–1002.
2. Burke, J. S., Byrne, G. E., Jr., and Rappaport, H.: Hairy cell leukemia (leukemic reticuloendotheliosis). Cancer 33:1399–1410, 1974.
3. Vykoupil, K. F., Thiele, J., and Georgii, A.: Hairy cell leukemia. Virchows Arch [Pathol Anat] 370:273–289, 1976.
4. Burke, J. S.: The value of the bone marrow biopsy in the diagnosis of hairy cell leukemia. Am J Clin Pathol 70:876–884, 1978.
5. Jansen, J., LeBien, T. W., and Kersey, J. H.: The phenotype of the neoplastic cells of hairy cell leukemia studied with monoclonal antibodies. Blood 59:609–614, 1982.

POORLY DIFFERENTIATED (SMALL-CLEAVED) LYMPHOCYTIC LYMPHOMA

The most common of the non-Hodgkin's lymphomas is that composed primarily or entirely of B-lymphocytes in the form designated as poorly differentiated or small-cleaved cells. This lesion represents approximately 50 per cent of cases in series of non-Hodgkin's lymphoma reported in the United States.[1–3] Although the tumor occurs in all decades of adult life it rarely develops in children.

When initially diagnosed the disease almost always involves lymph nodes, usually at multiple sites and in a symmetrical distribution above and below the diaphragm.[1–3] Despite this frequent dissemination, the bone marrow is affected in only about half the cases when the diagnosis is established.[4, 5] Remarkably, the telltale behavior of this lesion to form nodules that mimic germinal centers in lymph nodes and other involved tissues, which is evident in 60 to 90 per cent of cases, does not occur in the marrow. Nevertheless, the disposition of the tumor in the marrow

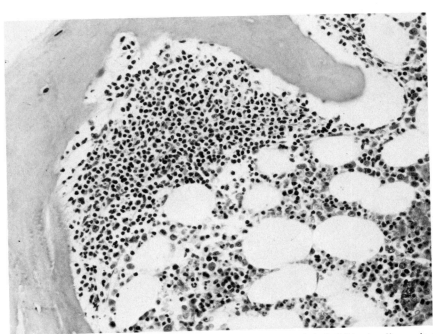

Figure 3–19. The paratrabecular propensity of these tumor cell aggregates is helpful in the diagnosis. 250×, H&E.

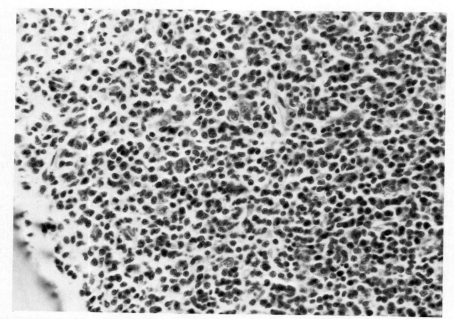

Figure 3–20. The marrow is diffusely involved in this case of poorly differentiated lymphocytic lymphoma. Only the cytological characteristics distinguish the disease from other lymphomas and leukemias. 250×, H&E.

is also idiosyncratic in that the cells have a propensity to cluster in a paratrabecular location (Fig. 3–19).[3, 4] This distribution may be the basis of the higher incidence of marrow disease detected by core biopsy as compared with aspiration. In fewer cases the marrow is diffusely infiltrated (Fig. 3–20).

Cytologically the tumor cell is best identified by its nucleus, which approximates the size of the well-differentiated lymphocyte and is elongated, indented, angulated, or twisted, but not round or convoluted (Fig. 3–21). The nuclear chromatin is clumped but not in blocks like that of the well-differentiated lym-

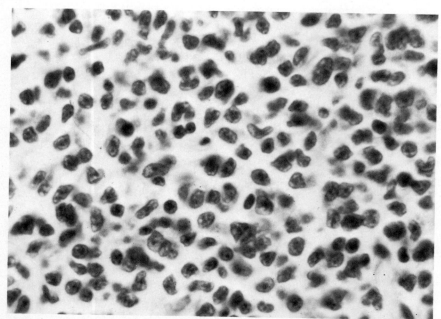

Figure 3–21. The irregular shape of the nuclei in conjunction with their relatively small size, clumped chromatin, and lack of mitotic activity distinguish this disease from most similar-appearing conditions. 1000×, H&E.

phocyte. Generally cytoplasm is difficult to visualize. Mitoses are rare.

About half of the cases with marrow infiltration have tumor cells in the peripheral blood, that is, lymphosarcoma cell leukemia.[5, 6] When these cells are identified in the blood it can be assumed that the marrow is involved.

The differential diagnostic considerations include well-differentiated lymphocytic lymphoma, large cell lymphoma, prolymphocytic leukemia, and hairy cell leukemia. The nuclear characteristics are usually sufficient to distinguish the poorly differentiated lymphocyte from the cells of the first three diseases even if the distribution of the cells is not helpful in a given case. In hairy cell leukemia when marrow involvement is focal the fine fibrillary network and perinuclear halo are the most useful differentiating features.

REFERENCES

1. Kim, H., and Dorfman, R. F.: Morphological studies of 84 untreated patients subjected to laparotomy for the staging of non-Hodgkin's lymphomas. Cancer 33:657–674, 1974.
2. Lotz, M. J., Chabner, B., DeVita, V. T., et al.: Pathological staging of 100 consecutive untreated patients with non-Hodgkin's lymphomas. Cancer 37:266–270, 1976.
3. Nathwani, B. N., Kim, H., Rappaport, H., et al.: Non-Hodgkin's lymphomas. Cancer 41:303–325, 1978.
4. Coller, B. S., Chabner, B. A., and Gralnick, H. R.: Frequencies and patterns of bone marrow involvement in non-Hodgkin's lymphomas. Am J Hematol 3:105–119, 1977.
5. Foucar, K., McKenna, R. W., Frizzera, G., et al.: Incidence and patterns of bone marrow and blood involvement by lymphoma in relationship to the Lukes-Collins classification. Blood 54:1417–1422, 1979.
6. Schnitzer, B., Loesel, L. S., and Reed, R. E.: Lymphosarcoma cell leukemia. Cancer 26:1082–1096, 1970.

LARGE CELL (HISTIOCYTIC) LYMPHOMA

Among the non-Hodgkin's lymphomas the large cell lymphoma, formerly designated as histiocytic lymphoma or reticulum cell sarcoma, has proved to be a most heterogeneous type morphologically and immunologically. The lesion constitutes approximately 25 per cent of the cases in series of non-Hodgkin's lymphoma reported in the United States.[1–3] In about one half of the cases the neoplastic cells are derived from B-lymphocytes and in 5 to 10 per cent from T-lymphocytes.[4] Currently about one third of the cases defy immunological classification. Only rarely do these "histiocytic" tumors arise from the monocyte-macrophage lineage to form true histiocytic lesions, currently designated *malignant histiocytosis*.

The reported frequency of marrow involvement ranges from 5 to 35 per cent.[5, 6] This wide variance probably reflects differences in cytological interpretation of the associated lymph node disease rather than a skewed geographical distribution. Tumors composed of mixtures of well-differentiated, poorly differentiated, and large lymphocytes may be classified in various ways by different observers. It is generally agreed, nevertheless, that marrow infiltration is less frequent in the large cell lymphoma than in the well- or poorly differentiated types. The presence of the large lymphocytes in the blood, that is, lymphosarcoma cell leukemia, is even less common.

Marrow involvement can be focal or widespread, but there is no paratrabecular preference. The tumor cells infiltrate between the fat cells in an interstitial fashion or form solid masses. The distinction between nodular and diffuse patterns made on the basis of lymph node histology is not possible in the marrow. Of the two cytological forms of large cell lymphoma, that composed of large non-cleaved cells is readily recognized by its large round to oval nuclei bearing one or more prominent nucleoli but little visible chromatin (Figs. 3–22A and B). Cytoplasm tends to be abundant, and cell borders are usually distinct. Mitoses are relatively common. Reticulin is increased but there is no collagen formation. The second cytological form, the cleaved type, consists of large lymphocytes distinguished by irregular, angulated, or dented nuclei with more visible chromatin but less visible nucleoli (Figs. 3–23A and B). Because the cell borders of these cells are not discernible, the nuclei appear to lie in a syncytium. Mitoses are less frequent than in the noncleaved form. In some cases the large lymphocytes are admixed with varying numbers of poorly and well-differentiated lymphocytes (Figs. 3–24A and B). When the large cells represent 25 per cent or more of the lymphoma cell population the lesion qualifies for this category. Distinct segregation of large and small cells in a lymphoma is unusual; when present, the lesion is designated *composite lymphoma*. This segregation can also be present in the marrow (Figs. 3–25A and B).

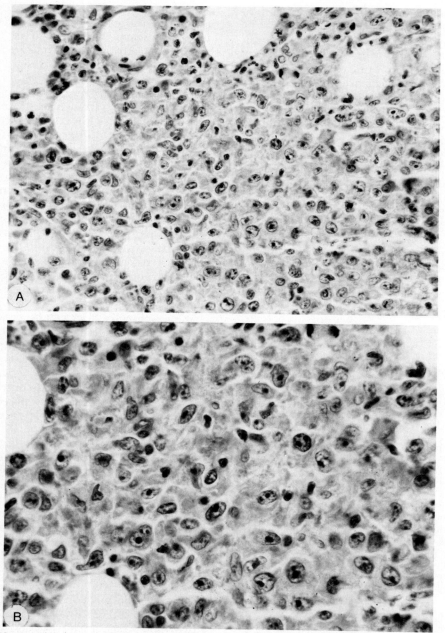

Figure 3–22. *A* and *B*. Cells with large round to oval vesicular nuclei containing prominent nucleoli are the identifying features of the large noncleaved type of lymphoma. Small to moderate amounts of cytoplasm may be present. 400× and 680×, H&E.

The immunoblastic lymphoma that had been classified as a large cell lymphoma is discussed elsewhere.

Differential diagnostic considerations include (1) poorly differentiated lymphocytic lymphoma, (2) Hodgkin's disease, and (3) metastatic carcinoma. The cleaved variety of large cell lymphoma may be simulated by poorly differentiated lymphocytic lymphoma when the distribution of the latter is diffuse rather than paratrabecular. The larger size of the nucleus and the presence of discerni-

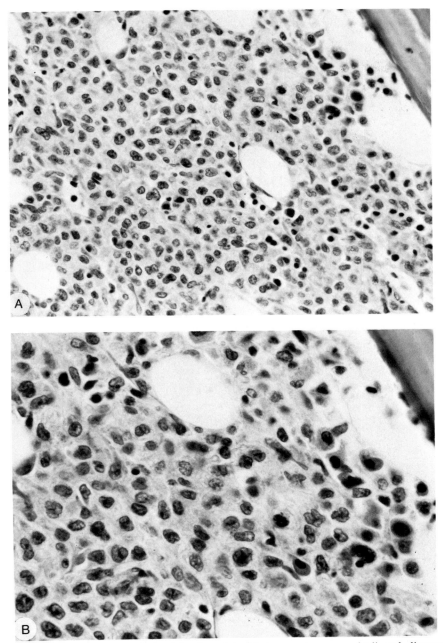

Figure 3–23. A and B. Large irregularly shaped nuclei with inconspicuous nucleoli and dispersed chromatin characterize the cells of the large cleaved type of lymphoma. The cytoplasm frequently appears to form a syncytium. 400× and 680×, H&E.

ble cytoplasm aid in distinguishing the former condition from the latter. As for Hodgkin's disease, the features of collagen fibrosis, heterogeneity of cell population, and Reed-Sternberg cells in various combinations serve to make the differentiation from large cell

lymphoma. Occasionally the small lymphocyte admixture in large cell lymphoma produces a heterogeneity suggestive of Hodgkin's disease. The lack of collagen and of Reed-Sternberg cells support the diagnosis of large cell lymphoma. An occasional case

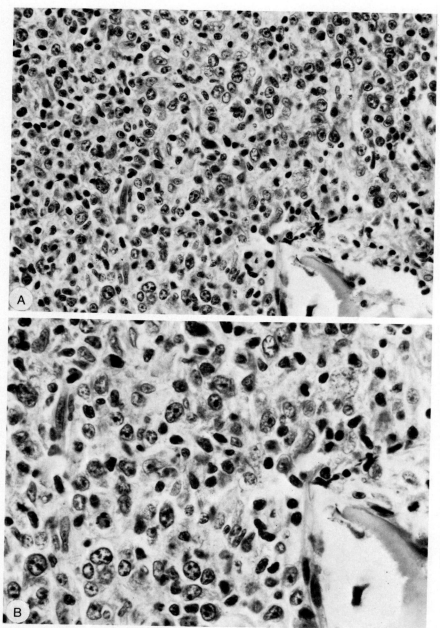

Figure 3–24. *A* and *B*. Large noncleaved lymphocytes and small cleaved lymphocytes mingle in almost equal numbers to produce the mixed type of lymphoma. 400× and 680×, H&E.

of Hodgkin's disease with abundant cohesive mononuclear "Hodgkin cells" may make diagnosis problematic. Usually there is a typical Reed-Sternberg cell present to settle the issue. Finally, cohesive groups of undifferentiated carcinoma cells may simulate large cell lymphoma. Unless there is an associated fibroplastic reaction, the only useful differen-

tiating feature, if present, is cytoplasmic vacuolization in carcinoma cells.

REFERENCES

1. Kim, H., and Dorfman, R. F.: Morphological studies of 84 untreated patients subjected to laparotomy for the staging of non-Hodgkin's lymphomas. Cancer 33:657–674, 1974.

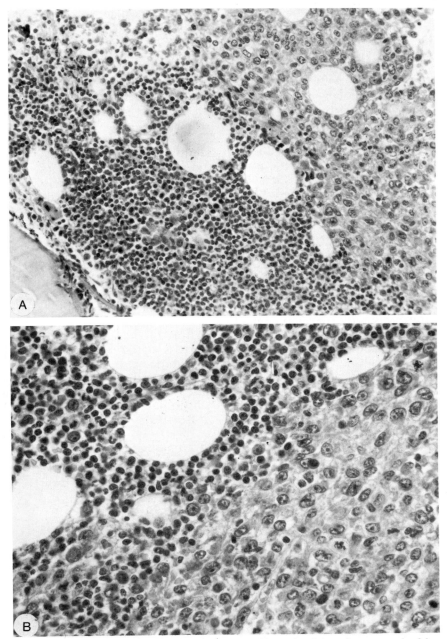

Figure 3–25. *A* and *B*. Distinctly segregated areas of well-differentiated lymphocytes and of large noncleaved lymphocytes in this composite lymphoma afford the opportunity to directly compare these two types of lymphocytes. 250× and 400×, H&E.

2. Lotz, M. J., Chabner, B., DeVita, V. T., et al.: Pathological staging of 100 consecutive untreated patients with non-Hodgkin's lymphomas. Cancer 37:266–270, 1976.
3. Nathwani, B. N., Kim, H., Rappaport, H., et al.: Non-Hodgkin's lymphomas. Cancer 41:303–325, 1978.
4. Berard, C. W., Jaffee, E. J., Braylan, R. C., et al.: Immunological aspects and pathology of the malignant lymphomas. Cancer 42:911–921, 1978.
5. Coller, B. S., Chabner, B. A., and Gralnick, H. R.: Frequencies and patterns of bone marrow involvement in non-Hodgkin's lymphomas. Am J Hematol 3:105–119, 1977.
6. Foucar, K., McKenna, R. W., Frizzera, G., et al.: Incidence and patterns of bone marrow and blood involvement by lymphoma in relationship to the Lukes-Collins classification. Blood 54:1417–1422, 1979.

IMMUNOBLASTIC LYMPHOMA

The elucidation of the immunological properties of the lymphocyte in its sundry forms eventually led to the recognition of lymphomas comprised of effector cells of either the B or the T cell lineages, that is, of immunoblasts. On the basis of readily demonstrable cytoplasmic gammaglobulin combined with characteristic morphology, the B-immunoblast and its lymphoma were identified. The T cell counterparts, on the other hand, have yet to receive universally accepted definitions.[1, 2] A restricted definition is based on the original description of the peripheral T cell lymphoma.[3] A broader view accepts all T cell lymphomas exclusive of cutaneous lymphomas and those consisting of lymphoblasts, well-differentiated lymphocytes, prolymphocytes, or hairy cells.[4, 5]

To date, primarily adults older than 50 have been reported to be affected by the disease. In some cases the development of immunoblastic lymphoma is preceded by diseases noted for immunological properties. These include Sjögren's syndrome, lupus erythematosus, rheumatoid arthritis, and angioimmunoblastic lymphadenopathy. Constitutional manifestations and peripheral lymph node enlargement are usually present, as may be hepatomegaly or splenomegaly. Abnormalities of peripheral blood cells are too inconstant to be of diagnostic value. A remarkable feature is the common occurrence of diffuse polyclonal hypergammaglobulinemia in the serum in cases of T-immunoblastic lymphoma and the occasional presence of monoclonal gammopathy in B-immunoblastic lymphoma.[4]

The marrow is involved in approximately 20 to 65 per cent of cases in the several small series reported.[6–10] Two distinctive marrow lesions can be recognized, that associated with T cell and that with the B cell lymphoma. Characteristically in the former type (Figs. 3–26A, B, and C), the lesions are focal and composed of a heterogeneous mixture of polymorphous lymphocytes commonly but not consistently admixed with histiocytes. The lymphocyte polymorphism is produced by variation in cell size and nuclear shape. The histiocytes usually have sufficient cytoplasm to produce an epithelioid appearance. Mature plasma cells and eosinophils are most obvious at the periphery of the foci and in the immediately surrounding marrow. The focality of the lesions is emphasized by the presence of an irregular stromal net of fibrils sometimes carrying a few capillaries or spindle-shaped stromal cells. By contrast, the B

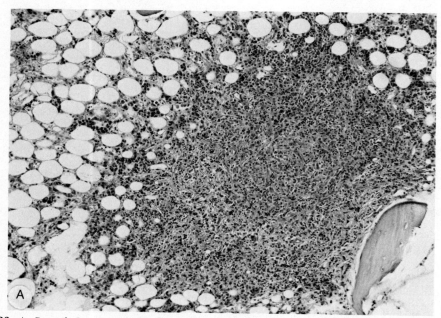

Figure 3–26. *A, B,* and *C.* Immunoblastic lymphoma, polymorphous variant. Lesions typically punctuate the marrow as more or less distinctly circumscribed foci. The heterogeneous lymphoid cell population is admixed with lesser numbers of bulky histiocytes distributed singly or in small clusters. Plasma cells and eosinophils are most notable at the periphery of the lesions. Elongated cells with spindly nuclei representing fibroblasts and endothelial cells in capillary channels complete the cytological inventory of this lesion. 100×, 250x and 680×, H&E.

Illustration continued on opposite page

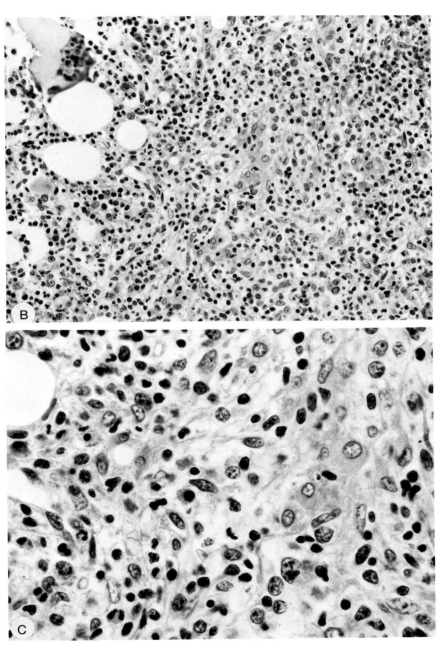

Figure 3–26. *Continued.*

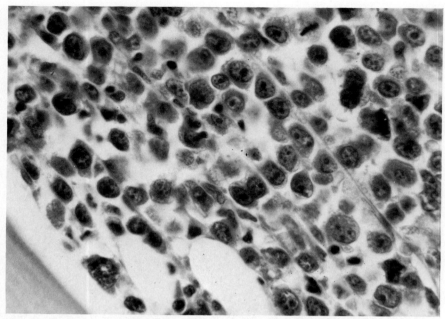

Figure 3–27. Immunoblastic lymphoma, plasmacytoid variant. In this lymphoma sheets of large transformed lymphocytes with large round nuclei carrying strikingly prominent, centrally located nucleoli and surrounded by rims of basophilic cytoplasm bear a clear resemblance to plasmablasts. 680×, H&E.

cell lesion is anatomically monotonous and serves as the morphological link between the large noncleaved lymphocytic lymphoma and the plasmablastic myeloma. The cell size and nucleus resemble the former condition, and the nucleus and cytoplasm resemble the latter (Fig. 3–27).

Differential diagnostic considerations include (1) Hodgkin's disease, (2) mixed lymphomas consisting of small cleaved and large lymphocytes with focal marrow involvement, (3) angioimmunoblastic lymphadenopathy, and (4) granulomatous reactions. Because of the potential variations in the features of each of these diseases the diagnosis of immunoblastic lymphoma in the marrow should be made only in conjunction with the diagnosis of lymph node disease.

REFERENCES

1. Neiman, R. S.: Immunoblastic sarcoma. Am J Surg Pathol 6:755–760, 1982.
2. Collins, R. D.: T-neoplasms. Am J Surg Pathol 6:745–754, 1982.
3. Waldron, J. A., Leech, J. H., Glick, A. D., et al.: Malignant lymphoma of peripheral T-lymphocyte origin. Cancer 40:1604–1617, 1977.
4. Maurer, R., Taylor, C. R., Parker, J. W., et al.: Immunoblastic sarcoma: Morphological criteria and the distinction of B and T cell types. Oncology 39:42–50, 1982.
5. Levine, A. M., Taylor, C. R., Schneider, D. R., et al.: Immunoblastic sarcoma of T-cell versus B-cell origin. Blood 58:52–61, 1981.
6. Burke, J. S., and Butler, J. J.: Malignant lymphoma with a high content of epithelioid histiocytes (Lennert's lymphoma). Am J Clin Pathol 66:1–9, 1976.
7. Nathwani, B. N., Rappaport, H., Moran, E. M., et al.: Malignant lymphoma arising in angioimmunoblastic lymphadenopathy. Cancer 41:578–606, 1978.
8. Kim, H., Jacobs, C., Warnke, R. A., et al.: Malignant lymphoma with a high content of epithelioid histiocytes. Cancer 41:620–635, 1978.
9. Palutke, M., Tabaczka, P., Weise, R. W., et al.: T-cell lymphomas of large cell type. Cancer 46:87–101, 1980.
10. Brisbane, J. U., Berman, L. D., and Neiman, R. J.: Peripheral T-cell lymphoma. Am J Clin Pathol 79:285–293, 1983.

ANGIOIMMUNOBLASTIC LYMPHADENOPATHY

This disease is currently viewed as a benign and generalized response of the immune system to extraneous agents such as drugs and viruses.[1, 2] Generalized or regional lymph node enlargement with a specific pathomorphology is an essential feature. The postulated immunological basis is reflected hema-

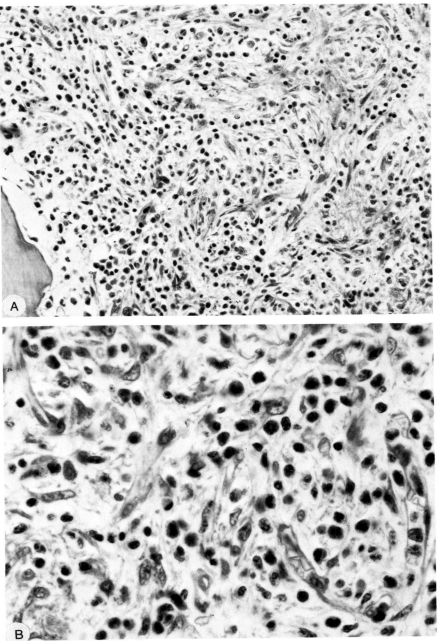

Figure 3–28. *A* and *B*. In this lesion the hematopoietic population consists of lymphoid cells and granulocytes. These are scattered through a haphazardly woven fibrillary mat containing spindly fibroblasts and delicate-appearing capillaries with prominent endothelial cells. 250× and 680×, H&E.

tologically by the frequent presence of Coombs' test–positive hemolytic anemia, immunocytophilia, lymphocytopenia, eosinophilia, and immune thrombocytopenia. Polyclonal hypergammaglobulinemia is also common. Marrow involvement has been demonstrated by core biopsy in 70 per cent of the cases.[3]

Current observations indicate that this disease can either remit completely or progress and evolve from a benign reaction to a lymphoma. Thus, in terms of hematopoietic cell behavior this disease may serve as a conceptual or even actual bridge between reactive hyperplasia and malignant proliferation, that is, a lymphodysplasia. The development of immunoblastic lymphoma in the marrow has been observed in approximately 20 per cent of cases showing the evolution to lymphoma in lymph nodes.[4]

The histopathology in the marrow core specimen has been clearly described.[3] Discrete or confluent lesions are distinguished from surrounding marrow by virtue of a decrease in cellularity, an increase in fibrous tissue, and a decrease or absence of fat cells (Figs. 3–28A and B). The cell population is heterogeneous, consisting of lymphocytes, plasma cells, immunocytes, and eosinophils. Groups of histiocytes are present occasionally but do not form granulomas. The intensity of the fibrosis varies from a delicate mesh to thick bands. Delicate capillaries and fibroblasts commonly traverse the lesions. The surrounding marrow may be normal or hypercellular but in the event of prior chemotherapy can be depleted of hematopoietic cells.

The principal differential diagnostic considerations are Hodgkin's disease and T-immunoblastic lymphoma. Reed-Sternberg cells or variants are the essential feature in differentiating Hodgkin's disease, since both diseases can be focal or diffuse in extent and polymorphous in composition. In immunoblastic lymphoma the lymphocyte population may comprise small and large and cleaved and noncleaved forms as well as immunoblasts. Confirmation of the marrow diagnosis on the basis of accompanying lymph node disease is obligatory in all three of these disorders.

REFERENCES

1. Frizzera, G., Moran, E. M., and Rappaport, H.: Angio-immunoblastic lymphadenopathy. Am J Med 59:803–818, 1975.
2. Lukes, R. J., and Tindle, B. H.: Immunoblastic lymphadenopathy. N Engl J Med 292:1–8, 1975.
3. Pangalis, G. A., Moran, E. M., and Rappaport, H.: Blood and bone marrow findings in angioimmunoblastic lymphadenopathy. Blood 51:71–83, 1978.
4. Nathwani, B. N., Rappaport, H., Moran, E. M., et al.: Malignant lymphoma arising in angioimmunoblastic lymphadenopathy. Cancer 41:578–606, 1978.

PLASMA CELL MYELOMA

The unrestricted proliferation and accumulation of a plasma cell monoclone in the marrow leads almost invariably to replacement of the normal hematopoietic cells and to destruction of the skeleton.[1] In most cases of myeloma the overwhelming number of plasma cells present in the marrow specimen constitutes sufficient evidence for the diagnosis. A concentration of plasma cells of less than 25 per cent, however, requires additional data to distinguish myeloma from reactive plasmacytosis. Most problematic cases can be resolved by the radiological demonstration of typical osteolytic lesions, by the finding of large numbers of plasma cells in a biopsy specimen from an osteolytic lesion, or by the presence of diagnostic levels of a monoclonal immunoglobulin or of its light chain moiety in the serum or urine.

The pelvic bones are among those most commonly affected by myeloma. Thus, the iliac crest biopsy can be a definitive procedure to establish the diagnosis. The core specimen is more valuable than the aspirated specimen, since the percentage of plasma cells as a function of total hematopoietic cell content and their distribution can be assessed better in a section of the core. Biopsy of the marrow is also a more sensitive method than x-ray examination for detection of myeloma, since mineralization of the bone must be reduced by about 50 per cent in order for lytic lesions to be visualized by x-ray examination.

In the marrow specimen several topographical features have been proposed as useful in differentiating myeloma from reactive plasmacytosis.[2, 3] Basically these features simply reflect the number of plasma cells that are present. In myeloma the plasma cells infiltrate between and progressively replace the fat cells as they occupy increasing amounts of the intertrabecular space. Unlike lymphoma, clearly defined cell clusters are unusual. By contrast, in reactive states such as chronic infections, chronic liver disease, and chronic rheumatoid arthritis, the plasma cells are largely restricted to the perivascular zone. This localization is vividly shown in the hypocellular phase marrow of acute myeloblastic leukemia following effective chemotherapy.

The character of the plasma cells is variable from case to case but usually uniform in a given case. In about one half of the cases the cells closely resemble well-differentiated plasma cells (Fig. 3–29). A diagnosis of myeloma based on morphology in these instances depends on an abundance of plasma cells in excess of 25 per cent of the hematopoietic cell content. In another one third of the cases the overly numerous plasma cells show fea-

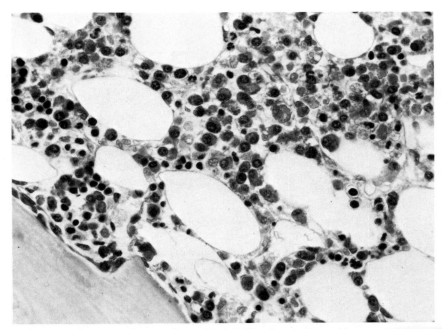

Figure 3–29. Myeloma with mature plasma cells randomly infiltrating the interstitium at a concentration exceeding 25 per cent. Cytologically these plasma cells are indistinguishable from those responding to an infectious or immunological stimulus. 400×, H&E.

tures of immaturity—enlarged cell size, pale basophilic cytoplasm, a centrally placed enlarged nucleus, and a nucleolus surrounded by dispersed chromatin (Fig. 3–30). These moderately differentiated cells are recognizable as plasma cells when they are present in sheets and clusters but individually can be confused with promyelocytes or basophilic normoblasts. In about 10 per cent of cases pleomorphism is pronounced, with many of the cells being large, multinucleated, or containing a very large eosinophilic nucleolus (Fig. 3–31). Multinuclearity is not specific for myeloma, but only rarely do plasma cells with more than two nuclei occur except in myeloma. Finally, in the few remaining cases plasma cells appear very immature, show mitotic activity, and may be misidentified as myeloblasts, lymphoblasts, or erythroblasts. Evidence of monoclonal immunoglobulin or light chain production is necessary to establish the diagnosis in these cases.

Many inclusions have been described in plasma cells, the first being the Russell body, and the most recent, the Dutcher body. All of these inclusions occur in reactive plasmacytosis as well as in myeloma and thus serve no useful purpose in the differential diagnosis.

The notorious ability of myeloma to de-stroy the skeleton is allegedly mediated by the production of an osteoclastic stimulating factor by the neoplastic plasma cells.[4] In the standard marrow core specimen osseous destruction can be manifested by loss of trabeculae, as indicated by an increased intertrabecular distance, by attenuated trabeculae, scalloped trabecular surfaces, or by isolated osteoclasts lying in resorption bays (Fig. 3–32). The latter were identified in 18 of 50 consecutive core specimens from cases of myeloma. Occasionally osteoblasts cover a trabecula, or the bone is coated by a thin layer of fibrous tissue.

Effective chemotherapy of myeloma is manifested in the marrow core specimen with features similar to those occurring in treated leukemia.

There are three potential sources of difficulty or error in establishing a diagnosis of myeloma: pronounced reactive plasmacytosis, the unusual nonsecretory myeloma, and benign monoclonal gammopathy. Application of the immunoperoxidase technique to the standard marrow core specimen can provide the deciding evidence in most of these cases by elucidating the character of the immunoglobulin in the plasma cells (Fig. 3–33).[5] Equivocal cases of reactive plasmacytosis can be clarified by the detection of both kappa

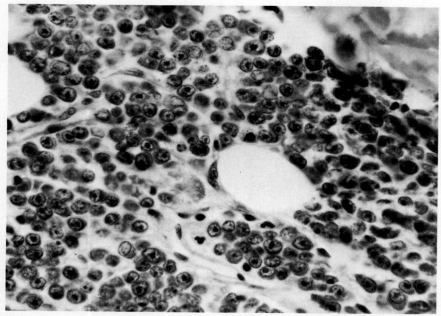

Figure 3–30. Myeloma with immature plasma cells or plasmablasts as evidenced by the vesicular nuclei bearing conspicuous nucleoli. Eccentricity of the nucleus, abundant cytoplasm, and a developed Golgi zone ("Hof") indicate progressive maturation in some cells. Any doubt concerning the identification of immature plasma cells may be resolved by use of the immunoperoxidase technique to demonstrate immunoglobulin. 525×, H&E.

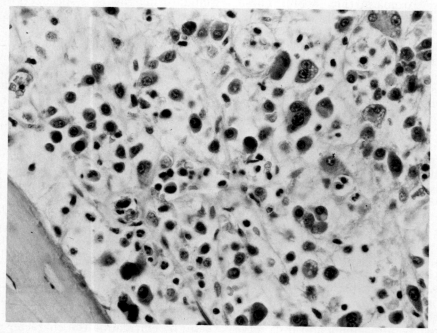

Figure 3–31. Myeloma with sparsely populated marrow after chemotherapy. A mixture of mature and immature and bi- and trinucleated plasma cells is present. 400×, H&E.

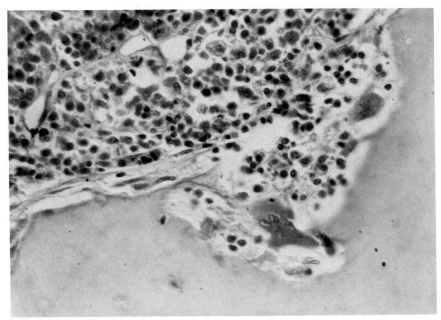

Figure 3–32. Osteoclast-mediated bone destruction in myeloma. The lesion may simulate osteodystrophy, but with rare exception there is no concomitant osteoblast activation in myeloma. The majority of plasma cells are mature. 250×, H&E.

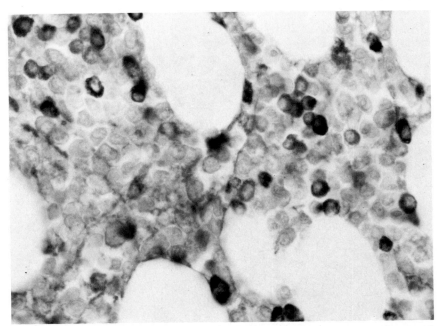

Figure 3–33. Immunoperoxidase demonstration of light chain moieties in reactive plasmacytosis reveal about equivalent amounts of both kappa and lambda chains, and thus with rare exceptions exclude the diagnosis of plasma cell myeloma. In this case the heavily stained cells contain kappa chain and the "shadow" plasma cells, as shown by a companion section, lambda chains. 680×, peroxidase antiperoxidase procedure.

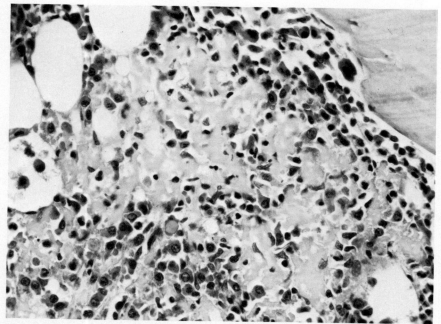

Figure 3–34. Myeloma complicated by amyloidosis. Note the Russell body in the left lower quadrant and the bone trabecula with an irregular surface and an adjacent osteoclast in the right upper quadrant. 400×, H&E.

and lambda light chains in the plasma cell population. This rule is rarely if ever violated. In the nonsecretory myeloma the technique is valuable for establishing the monoclonal nature of the plasma cell population and for defining the immunoglobulin produced. Finally, in benign monoclonal gammopathy an increase in the number of plasma cells to as much as 20 per cent of the marrow cell population can be associated with the

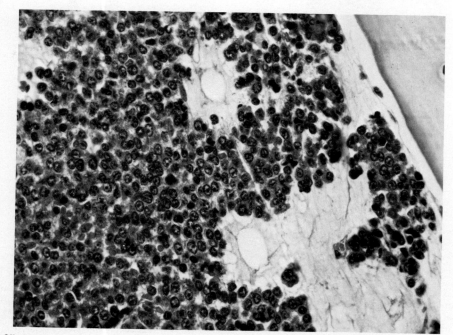

Figure 3–35. Myeloma accompanied by serous atrophy of fat, which should be distinguished from amyloidosis. 400×, H&E.

immunoglobulinemia. In the past the problem has been clarified only by longitudinal study of the patient. Recently it has been reported that as in reactive plasmacytosis more than one class of immunoglobulin and both kappa and lamba light chains are present in the plasma cell population in these cases.[3]

Amyloidosis, the uncommon complication of myeloma, is discussed elsewhere (Fig. 3–34). This condition can be simulated by serous atrophy of residual fat cells (Fig. 3–35).

REFERENCES

1. Bergsagel, D. E.: Plasma cell myeloma. *In* Williams, W. J., Beutler, E., Erslev, A. J., and Lichtman, M. A. (eds.): Hematology. New York, McGraw-Hill, 1983, pp. 1078–1104.
2. Hyun, B. H., Kwa, D., Gabaldon, H., et al.: Reactive plasmacytic lesions of the bone marrow. Am J Clin Pathol 65:921–928, 1976.
3. Bartl, R., Frisch, B., Burkhardt, R., et al.: Bone marrow histology in myeloma: Its importance in diagnosis, prognosis, classification and staging. Br J Haematol 51:361–375, 1982.
4. Mundy, G. R., Raisz, L. G., Cooper, R. A., et al.: Evidence for the secretion of an osteoclast stimulating factor in myeloma. N Engl J Med 291:1041–1046, 1974.
5. Pinkus, G. S., and Said, J. W.: Specific identification of intracellular immunoglobulin in paraffin sections of multiple myeloma and macroglobulinemia using an immunoperoxidase technique. Am J Pathol 87:47–58, 1977.

WALDENSTRÖM'S MACROGLOBULINEMIA

In its fully developed state this disease characteristically displays features of both lymphoma and myeloma—the lymph node enlargement and hepatosplenomegaly of the former and the monoclonal immunoglobulinemia of the latter.[1] Theoretically this disparate combination may reflect a midcourse arrest in the conversion of a lymphocyte monoclone to one of plasma cells. The excessive production of monoclonal IgM is the hallmark of the disease and customarily is a requisite for the diagnosis.

In the marrow core section sheets or clusters of lymphoid cells displace to varying degrees the normal hematopoietic cells. The neoplastic cells are, in varying proportions, lymphocytes, plasma cells, and hybrid cells having the nucleus of a lymphocyte and the cytoplasm of a plasma cell, the so-called *lymphoplasma cell* (Fig. 3–36). The latter is more

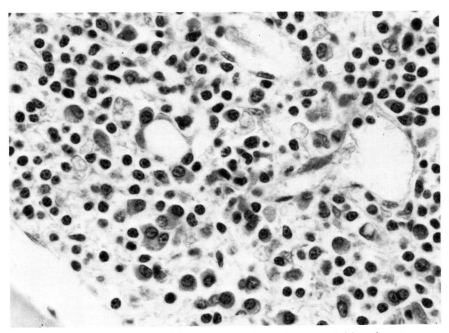

Figure 3–36. A heterogeneous population of plasma cells and well-differentiated lymphocytes occupy the marrow in this case. Lymphoplasma cells, though commonly present, are difficult to recognize in sections. There is an apparent intranuclear inclusion in a single cell in the right lower quadrant and a cell distended with large cytoplasmic vacuoles in the left upper quadrant. 680×, H&E.

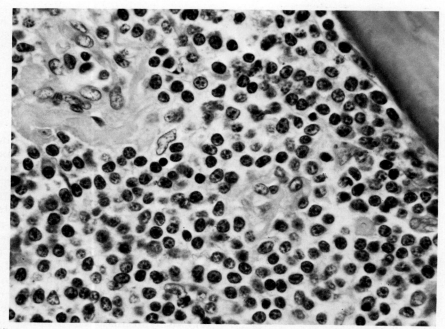

Figure 3–37. Intercellular deposit of a hyaline amorphous substance occurs in about half the cases. 680×, H&E.

accurately identified in smears than in marrow sections. Any of the cellular inclusions found in plasma cell myeloma may be present. Amorphous hyaline material is deposited among the lymphoid cells in about one half of the cases (Fig. 3–37). This periodic acid-Schiff–positive material has properties of IgM rather than of amyloid.[2, 3] The trabecular bone is normal.

The diagnosis of Waldenström's macroglobulinemia may in some cases revolve around the defining characteristics employed. In its classic form the disease is manifested by increased serum levels of IgM, increased numbers of lymphocytes, plasma cells, and lymphoplasma cells in the marrow, and inconstantly by anemia, bleeding, hyperviscosity of the blood, and enlargement of lymph nodes, liver, and spleen.[1] Reports in which the definition is based only on serum Ig phenotype state that the marrow features are inconstant.[2] Other reports claim that the disease can be associated with monoclonal IgG or IgA rather than IgM.[4] Yet other reports describe typical cases of plasma cell myeloma including bone destruction associated with IgM macroglobulinemia.[5] In the context of B-lymphocyte physiology these uncommon variations can be expected and rationalized. They are probably best viewed as variant forms of lymphocytic lymphoma or plasma cell myelomas as, in fact, can Waldenström's macroglobulinemia.

In evaluating the marrow core section, differential diagnostic considerations include chronic lymphocytic leukemia and well-differentiated lymphocytic lymphoma, plasma cell myeloma, and reactive plasmacytosis or lymphocytosis. Lymphocytes, plasma cells, and lymphoplasma cells in an aggregate sum exceeding 25 per cent are almost assuredly a neoplastic proliferation rather than a reaction. The demonstration of idiotypic IgM production by standard procedures including cellular immunoperoxidase substantiates not only the diagnosis of neoplasia but also of macroglobulinemia.[6]

REFERENCES

1. Bergsagel, D. E.: Macroglobulinemia. *In* Williams, W. J., Beutler, E., Erslev, A. J., and Lichtman, M. A. (eds.): Hematology. New York, McGraw-Hill, 1983, pp. 1104–1109.
2. Rywlin, A. M., Civantos, F., Ortega, R. S., et al.: Bone marrow histology in monoclonal macroglobulinemia. Am J Clin Pathol 63:769–778, 1975.
3. Case Records of the Massachusetts General Hospital (case 42-1982). N Engl J Med 307:1065–1073, 1982.

4. Tursz, T., Brouet, J. C., Flandrin, G., et al.: Clinical and pathological features of Waldenström's macroglobulinemia in seven patients with serum monoclonal IgG or IgA. Am J Med 63:499–502, 1977.
5. Zarrabi, M. H., Stark, R. S., Kane P., et al.: IgM myeloma, a distinct entity in the spectrum of B-cell neoplasia. Am J Clin Pathol 75:1–10, 1981.
6. Pinkus, G. S., and Said, J. W. Specific identification of intracellular immunoglobulin in paraffin sections of multiple myeloma and macroglobulinemia using an immunoperoxidase technique. Am J Pathol 87:47–58, 1977.

AMYLOIDOSIS

The formation of amyloid in the marrow appears to be an uncommon event. According to current concepts, amyloid is formed by the conversion of either selected immunoglobulin light chain fragments or the non-immunoglobulin A-protein to a fibrillar product, which in combination with a glycoprotein is deposited on a receptive tissue component such as reticulin.[1, 2] The unique β-pleated sheet structure of the resultant fibrils appears to be the basis of the specific reaction pattern with Congo Red dye—a red color in direct light and green birefringence in polarized light. Light chain fragments serve as the source of the fibrillar product in primary and in myeloma-associated amyloidosis, while the A-protein is the source in the secondary forms and in certain heredofamilial types.

Histological examination is essential to establish the diagnosis of amyloidosis, and the marrow core biopsy has proved to be of value.[3] In primary amyloidosis the marrow is involved in about 50 per cent of cases. In myeloma, in which about 10 per cent of the cases develop amyloidosis, the marrow contains the amyloid in about 40 per cent of cases. The frequency in the secondary and heredofamilial forms is difficult to ascertain.

Amyloid in the marrow may be deposited within the walls of sinusoids or small vessels (Figs. 3–38 and 3–39), or in the stroma surrounding and engulfing hematopoietic cells and fat cells (Fig. 3–39). As in other tissues, the amyloid stained with hematoxylin and eosin has the smooth, amorphous, pink appearance of a hyaline substance. The specific reactions with Congo Red dye verifies the presence of amyloid. The use of other staining reactions and the distinction between amyloid and paramyloid are of doubtful value. Amyloid from an immunoglobulin light chain can be distinguished from that derived from A-protein by permanganate oxidation preceding Congo Red dye staining.[4] Only amyloid from immunoglobulin is resistant to oxidative destruction.

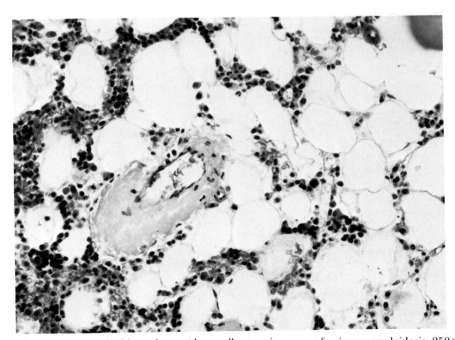

Figure 3–38. Amyloid deposited in and around a small artery in a case of primary amyloidosis. 250×, H&E.

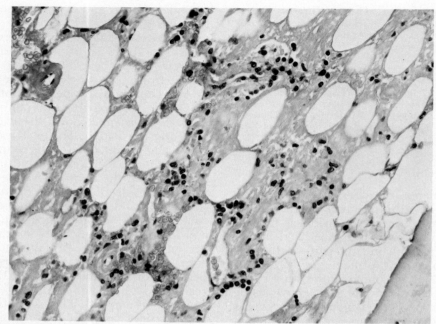

Figure 3–39. Amyloid permeating between the fat cells and enveloping the few remaining plasma cells in this case of plasma cell myeloma complicated by amyloidosis. A capillary-sized vessel in the left upper quadrant is also involved. This interstitial disposition of amyloid in the marrow should not be confused with serous atrophy of fat, which may on occasion be associated with plasma cell myeloma. 250×, H&E.

REFERENCES

1. Franklin, E. C.: Amyloidosis. *In* Williams, W. J., Beutler, E., Erslev, A. J., and Lichtman, M. A. (eds.): Hematology. New York, McGraw-Hill, 1983, pp. 1112–1118.
2. Glenner, G. G.: Amyloid deposits and amyloidosis. N Engl J Med 302:1283–1292 and 1333–1343, 1980.
3. Krause, J. R.: Value of bone marrow biopsy in the diagnosis of amyloidosis. South Med J 70:1072–1074, 1977.
4. van Rijswijk, M. H., and van Heusden, C. W. G. J.: The potassium permanganate method. Am J Pathol 97:43–54, 1979.

4

HODGKIN'S DISEASE

Hodgkin's disease rarely, if ever, originates in the bone marrow. Yet most patients with the disease eventually have marrow involvement.[1, 2] Spread to the marrow in some cases is caused by direct extension from affected lymph nodes or other tissue adjacent to the bone but far more commonly occurs by hematogenous dissemination. The routes followed from distant involved lymph nodes to the marrow have been postulated by Kaplan.[3] Since the marrow lacks lymphatic channels, entry of the malignant cells into the bloodstream is a requisite for marrow metastasis. Where this invasion occurs is uncertain, but the spleen or lymphatic-hematic junctions, such as the thoracic·duct, are probable sites. Currently marrow deposits in core biopsy specimens are demonstrated in about 10 per cent of cases before treatment is instituted.[4–6] They occur most commonly in conjunction with lymph node disease of the lymphocyte depletion type, less frequently in the mixed and nodular sclerosis forms, and rarely in lymphocyte predominance disease. Since the disease is usually not generalized in the marrow, as can be expected in a leukemia, biopsy of both iliac crests is recommended. Aspirates of marrow are rarely, if ever, useful in demonstrating the disease.[2, 7, 8]

The histopathology of Hodgkin's disease in marrow core specimens has been described in several reports.[4–6] Emphasis is placed on the heterogeneity of the features and the diligence required to find diagnostic Reed-Sternberg cells. Diagnostic cells cannot be identified in all cases in which other features suggest the presence of the disease. Regardless of whether the features are typical or not, it is inadvisable to base the diagnosis of Hodgkin's disease solely on a marrow core specimen.

The marrow lesions may be focal but more commonly extend between and surround the bone trabeculae. Despite the variety of features that can be present, the lesions are usefully evaluated in terms of cellularity, frequency of malignant cells, and abundance of collagen. Three categories can be recognized: cellular, fibrocellular, and fibrotic. Cellular lesions consist principally of benign histiocytes, of well-differentiated lymphocytes, or a mixture of both. Reed-Sternberg cells or their variants are variable in number (Figs. 4–1 and 4–2). Fibrous tissue is limited to a fine reticular network. In fibrocellular lesions, all of the ancillary cells making up the cellular environment of Hodgkin's disease are present in varying numbers but fibroblasts and collagen are conspicuous background features (Figs. 4–3 and 4–4). Reed-Sternberg cells and variants can range from undetectable to readily evident. In fibrotic lesions the ancillary and malignant cells are all but overshadowed by the abundance of fibroblasts and collagen (Fig. 4–5). The collagen may have a swirling or herring bone pattern.

The more cellular lesions generally occur in patients with nodular sclerosis or mixed cellularity type of lymph node disease, whereas the more fibrotic deposits are more common with the lymphocyte depletion type. The fibrotic lesion is most liable to misinterpretation when Reed-Sternberg cells cannot be found, and the diagnosis of Hodgkin's disease has not been established on the basis of lymph node pathology. Nonspecific fibrosis or chronic primary myelofibrosis is the usual errant diagnosis. The more cellular lesions may be mistaken for large cell, mixed lymphocytic, or immunoblastic lymphoma. Isolated small foci can mimic angioimmunoblastic lymphadenopathy.

Marrow not involved in the Hodgkin's dis-

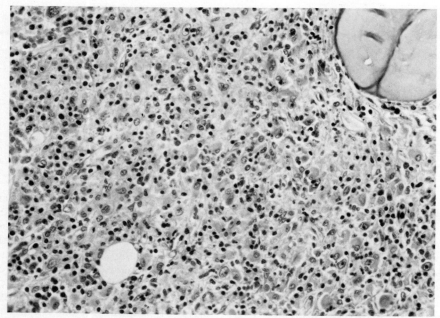

Figure 4–1. A cellular form of marrow disease in a case of Hodgkin's disease of the mixed cellularity type in a lymph node. Only a single Reed-Sternberg cell and a few mononuclear variants are present among the associated ancillary cells, the majority of which are small lymphocytes and histiocytes. 250×, (H&E).

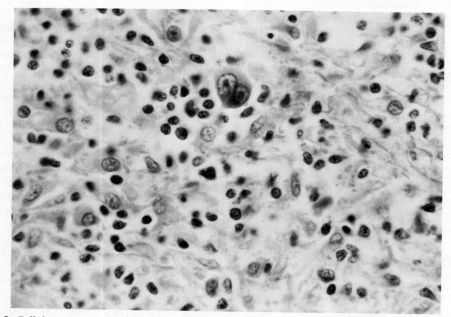

Figure 4–2. Cellular marrow disease in a case of Hodgkin's disease of the lymphocyte predominance type in a lymph node. A mixture of well-differentiated lymphocytes and bland-appearing histiocytes surround the lone Reed-Sternberg cell. 680×, H&E.

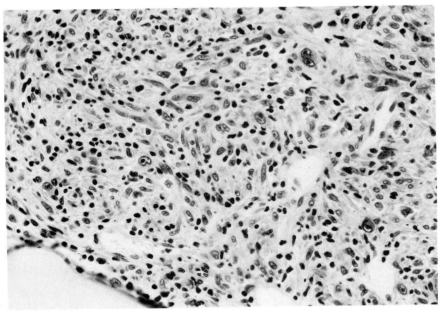

Figure 4–3. Marrow disease of the fibrocellular type in a case with nodal disease of the mixed cellularity type. Spindly fibroblasts and small amounts of collagen pervade the small lymphocytes and the isolated Reed-Sternberg cell and mononuclear variants. 325×, H&E.

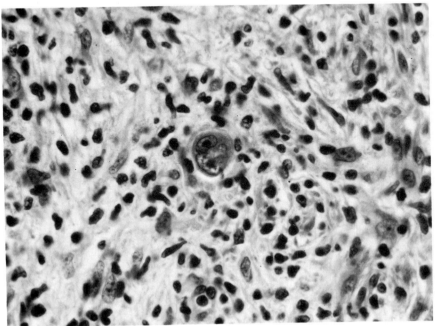

Figure 4–4. Fibrocellular marrow disease in a case of Hodgkin's disease of the nodular sclerosis type in a lymph node. Fibrosis is a more prominent background feature for the cellular population, which includes a Reed-Sternberg cell. 680×, H&E.

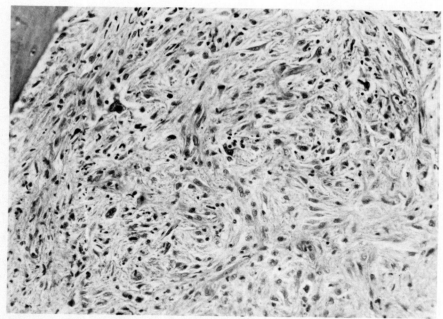

Figure 4–5. Fibrotic marrow disease in a case of Hodgkin's disease of the lymphocyte-depleted type in a lymph node. Few if any lymphocytes or histiocytes can be detected among the fibroblasts and collagen in which there are occasional distorted mononuclear variant cells. 250×, H&E.

ease may be normal or show granulocytic hyperplasia with or without an increase in megakaryocytes. Occasionally small isolated aggregates of well-differentiated lymphocytes are present.

Additional features that can be present are focal necrosis (Fig. 4–6) and angiogenesis.

These have been reported to occur especially after treatment[5, 6] but can also precede it. Better evidence in the marrow of effective therapy is either focal cellular depletion in affected sites (Fig. 4–7) or no evidence of residual disease.

As have been observed in the liver and

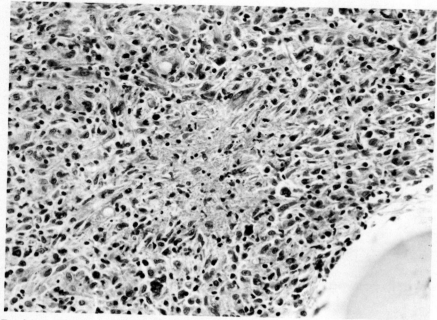

Figure 4–6. Focal necrosis in a case with cellular marrow disease and mixed cellularity nodal disease. 250×, H&E.

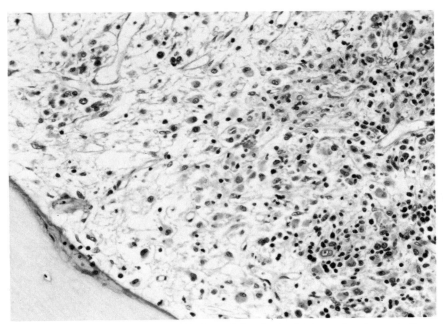

Figure 4–7. After chemotherapy in this case with the cellular form of marrow involvement, the marrow is only partially cleansed of disease. Monitoring the effectiveness of therapy by successive core biopsy is necessary in a case with marrow disease. 250×, H&E.

spleen, nonnecrotizing granulomas also occur in the marrow in Hodgkin's disease.[5, 6] They consist of clusters of histiocytes, some or all of which may be converted to epithe-

lioid cells or to giant cells (Figs. 4–8 and 4–9). The granulomas can exist either as isolated lesions or in association with the Hodgkin's disease. Cultures and histological stains for

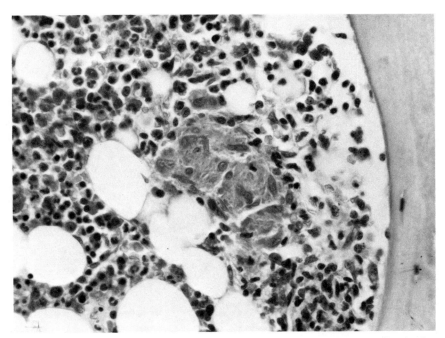

Figure 4–8. An isolated small cluster of epithelioid histiocytes was the only abnormality in the marrow after treatment of this case of Hodgkin's disease. Two years earlier the patient had lymphocyte-depleted nodal disease with a fibrotic type of marrow. 400×, H&E.

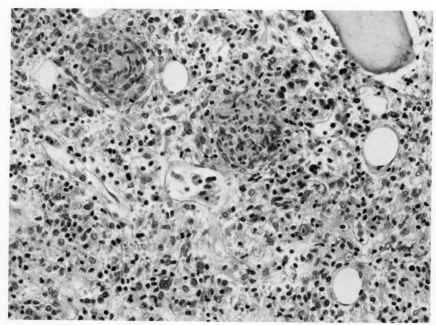

Figure 4–9. Conventional granulomas in the marrow accompany the cellular form of marrow involvement in this case of Hodgkin's disease of the mixed cellularity type. 250×, H&E.

microorganisms must be done before presuming they are noninfective. More common than granulomas and usually found in the cellular and fibrocellular lesions are rings of histiocytes surrounding optically clear spaces (Figs. 4–9 and 4–10). These histiocytic rings

bear no resemblance to lipogranulomas, nor do they appear to be a stage in granuloma formation. While their presence cannot be consistently correlated with prior lipoidal lymphangiography, chemotherapy, or radiation, they may be related to injection or

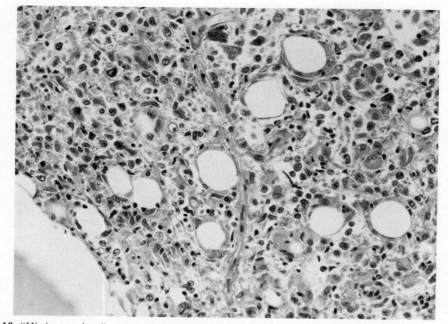

Figure 4–10. "Histiocyte rings" among the ancillary cells in a case of Hodgkin's disease of the mixed cellularity type, with cellular marrow disease. The rings are less conspicuous in Figure 4–9, which was obtained from a different case. 250×, H&E.

ıngestion of lipid compounds, as has been advocated for the granuloma.[9]

Since the initial diagnosis of Hodgkin's disease should rarely, if ever, be based solely on the pathology present in a marrow core specimen, differential diagnostic considerations concern only whether given features are indicative of the disease, are ancillary, or are consequent to treatment. Granulomas, isolated lymphocyte aggregates, and granulocytic hyperplasia with or without megakaryocytic hyperplasia are ancillary features and are not considered to be evidence of Hodgkin's disease in the marrow. On the other hand, foci of collagen fibrosis with few or many mononuclear Hodgkin's cells and varying numbers of lymphocytes, plasma cells, and granulocytes but without Reed-Sternberg cells should be diagnosed as Hodgkin's disease in the marrow with the provision that the definitive diagnosis has been established previously. This view has been expressed by others.[10] The development of myelodysplasia, acute myeloblastic leukemia, or lymphoma as an aftermath of therapy for Hodgkin's disease can also be expressed in the marrow and complicate the interpretation of the core specimen.[11, 12]

REFERENCES

1. Thomas, L. B., and Berard, C. W.: Hodgkin's disease: Relationship of histopathologic type at diagnosis to clinical parameters and to histopathological progression and anatomical distribution at autopsy. *In* Akazaki, K., Rappaport, H., Berard, C. W., Bennett, J. M., and Ishikawa, E. (eds.): Gann Monograph on Cancer Research 15. Tokyo, University of Tokyo Press, 1973, pp. 253–273.

2. Han, T., Stutzman, L., and Roque, A. L.: Bone marrow biopsy in Hodgkin's disease and other neoplastic diseases. JAMA 217:1239–1241, 1971.

3. Kaplan, H. S.: Hodgkin's Disease. Cambridge, Harvard University Press. 1980.

4. Myers, C. E., Chabner, B. A., DeVita, V. T., et al.: Bone marrow involvement in Hodgkin's disease: Pathology and response to MOPP chemotherapy. Blood 44:197–204, 1974.

5. O'Carroll, D. I., McKenna, R. W., and Brunning, R. D.: Bone marrow manifestations of Hodgkin's disease. Cancer 38:1717–1728, 1976.

6. Bartl, R., Frisch, B., Burkhardt, R., et al.: Assessment of bone marrow histology in Hodgkin's disease. Correlation with clinical factors. Br J Haematol 51:345–360, 1982.

7. Grann, V., Pool, J. L., and Mayer, K.: Comparative study of bone marrow aspiration and biopsy in patients with neoplastic disease. Cancer 19:1898–1900, 1966.

8. Webb, D. I., Ubogy, G., and Silver, R. T.: Importance of bone marrow biopsy in the clinical staging of Hodgkin's disease. Cancer 26:313–317, 1970.

9. Pak, H. Y., and Friedman, N. B.: Pseudosarcoid granulomas in Hodgkin's disease. Hum Pathol 12:832–837, 1981.

10. Lee, R. E., and Ellis, L. D.: Histopathologic and clinical findings in Hodgkin's disease of the bone marrow. Am J Clin Pathol 65:268, 1976.

11. Krikorian, J. G., Burke, J. S., Rosenberg, S. A., et al.: Occurrence of non-Hodgkin's lymphoma after therapy for Hodgkin's disease. N Engl J Med 300:452–458, 1979.

12. Pedersen-Bjergaard, J., and Larsen, S. O.: Incidence of acute nonlymphocytic leukemia, preleukemia, and acute myeloproliferative syndrome up to 10 years after treatment of Hodgkin's disease. N Engl J Med 307:965–971, 1982.

5

HISTIOCYTE PROLIFERATIVE DISEASES

CONCEPT AND SCOPE

The many faces, functions, and abodes of the histiocyte have greatly complicated its recognition. As a result, the definition and delineation of reactions, hyperplasias, and neoplasias arising from this cell, its precursors, and its progeny have been unduly difficult to make.[1] On the one hand, the histiocyte is related to the monocyte, and recently this ancestral chain has been traced back to the myeloblast.[2] On the other hand, with maturation and dispersion to sites throughout the body where interaction with animate and inanimate materials may occur, the histiocyte has shown the ability to assume a dozen different guises to which an equal number of names have been assigned. The most popular among these are *macrophage*, with a variety of modifying adjectives, and *mononuclear phagocyte*. The result of this seemingly endless variety is that benign and malignant or reactive and neoplastic hematopoietic diseases stemming from the histiocyte have probably been misdiagnosed and received more names than most others in hematology.

Among the multiplicity of roles currently assigned to the histocyte, the inflammatory reaction, the immune response, and the storage and degradation of cells and products are the most clearly defined.[3] Defects in one or more of these tasks may be evident in some of the diseases in this group. These defects are best defined for the inherited single enzyme storage diseases[4, 5] and most recently have been described for histiocytosis X.[6]

The terminology used here is based on the recognized relation between the monocyte and the macrophage as well as the time-honored use of the term "histiocyte." The latter is employed to indicate the developmental stage beyond the monocyte and to include the macrophage as a morphologic subset recognized by its cytoplasmic content of phagocytized structures or derived products.

Four diseases or groups of diseases have sufficient impact on the marrow to be considered. Two are viewed as autochthonous neoplasms—*histiocytosis X* and *malignant histiocytosis*—and two as reactions—*storage histiocytosis* and *benign reactive histiocytosis*. Histiocytosis X is presented as a group of disorders because of the evidence that the various syndromes all arise from the specialized histiocyte, the *Langerhans' cell*.[7] Some forms such as the unifocal eosinophilic granuloma can be considered comparable to the adenoma among the epithelial neoplasms and others such as Letterer-Siwe disease as analogous to the carcinoma. The contention that histiocytosis X is not a neoplasm because the lesion is morphologically heterogeneous is a specious argument;[6] for example, the histology of Hodgkin's disease may be considered. The storage histiocytoses are considered benign hyperplasias that reflect a need to deal with the normal catabolic requirement in disposing of effete cells in the face of a critical enzyme deficiency. Albeit serious clinically, benign reactive histiocytosis is so designated because it is a response comparable to the inflammatory response of the neutrophil and not a neoplasm. Its recognition as an entity stems from the use of highly effective immunosuppressive and cytotoxic chemotherapy.[8] The disease has also occurred in other settings, most frequently with severe viral infections.[8, 9]

Logically, several other diseases could be included in this group. The heritable diseases, chronic granulomatous disease and Chediak-Higashi syndrome, are candidates, since the monocyte-macrophage lineage is affected although the impaired neutrophil function is clinically more serious. That both lineages are involved was predictable from current theory of a common progenitor for these cells.[1] Granulomatous inflammation can also be included as a reactive histiocytosis, although this condition is localized in the sense of forming discrete cell clusters rather than sheets or a diffuse dispersion of cells. In theory the monocytic and myelomonocytic leukemias could also be included here.[1] However, they are more suitably treated as myeloproliferative diseases. Finally, Hodgkin's disease could be placed in this group.[10]

REFERENCES

1. Groopman, J. E., and Golde, D. W.: The histiocytic disorders: A pathophysiologic analysis. Ann Intern Med 94:95–107, 1981.
2. Koeffler, H. P., Bar-Eli, M., and Territo, M.: Phorbol diester-induced macrophage differentiation of leukemia blasts from patients with human myelogenous leukemia. J Clin Invest 66:1101–1108, 1980.
3. Lasser, A.: The mononuclear phagocytic system: A review. Hum Pathol 14:108–126, 1983.
4. Brady, R. O., and Barranger, J. A.: Glucosylceramide lipidosis: Gaucher's disease. *In* Stanbury, J. B., Wyngaarden, J. B., Fredrickson, D. S., Goldstein, J. L., and Brown, M. S. (eds.): The Metabolic Basis of Inherited Diseases. 5th ed. New York, McGraw-Hill, 1983, pp. 842–856.
5. Brady, R. O.: Sphingomyelin lipidosis: Niemann-Pick's disease. *In* Stanbury, J. G., Wyngaarden, J. B., Fredrickson, D. S., Goldstein, J. L., and Brown, M. S. (eds.): The Metabolic Basis of Inherited Diseases. 5th ed. New York, McGraw-Hill, 1983, pp. 831–841.
6. Osband, M. E., Lipton, J. M., Lavin, P., et al.: Histiocytosis-X: Demonstration of abnormal immunity, T-cell histamine H_2 receptor deficiency, and successful treatment with thymic extract. N Engl J Med 304:146–153, 1981.
7. Nezelof, C.: Histiocytosis X: A histological and histogenetic study. *In* Rosenberg, H. S., and Bernstein, J. (eds.): Perspectives in Pediatric Pathology. Vol. 5. New York, Masson Publishing USA, Inc., 1979, pp. 153–178.
8. Risdall, R. J., McKenna, R. W., Nesbit, M. E., et al.: Virus-associated hemophagocytic syndrome. Cancer 44:993–1002, 1979.
9. Chandra, P., Chaudbery, S. A., Rosner, F., et al.: Transient histiocytosis with striking phagocytosis of platelets, leukocytes, and erythrocytes. Arch Intern Med 135:989–991, 1975.
10. Kaplan, H. S.: Hodgkin's disease: Unfolding concepts concerning its nature, management and prognosis. Cancer 45:2439–2474, 1980.

MALIGNANT HISTIOCYTOSIS

More precise and reliable identification of all hematopoietic cells and their neoplasias, especially with respect to the lymphocyte, has led with increasing frequency to the proper recognition of the malignant histiocyte in all of its variations and permutations. Classically, malignant histiocytic disease is described as an acute febrile rapidly devastating illness with hepatosplenomegaly and lymph node enlargement occurring in children and is known as *histiocytic medullary reticulosis.* Currently, the disease is recognized as also occurring as an isolated splenomegaly, localized lymph node enlargement, or skin rash in all age groups, and is more widely known as *malignant histiocytosis.*[1–4]

In the blood pancytopenia or selective cytopenia is usually present. This has been attributed to phagocytosis by the better differentiated members among the neoplastic histiocytes. More importantly for diagnostic purposes, abnormal histiocytes, including blast cells and atypical monocytoid cells, circulate in the peripheral blood in as many as 90 per cent of cases; in almost half the cases these cells consist of over 10 per cent of the circulating white cells.[5]

Many reports minimize the value of marrow examination for aid in diagnosis. Yet in one recently recorded series all of 12 cases had abnormal histiocytes in the marrow aspirate, and in all but two of the cases 10 per cent or more of the marrow cells were abnormal histiocytes.[5] Similar opinions have been expressed about the marrow core biopsy. In the same series, all but one of seven cases so examined showed the disease in the core specimen.

The cellularity of the core specimen is variable, as is the proportion of normoblasts, developing granulocytes, and megakaryocytes. Owing to ease of recognition the most critical diagnostic feature is the phagocytizing histiocyte containing one or more ingested cells. Most commonly these ingested cells are red cells or normoblasts and less commonly granulocytes, lymphocytes, or platelets. Admixed with the phagocytizing cells and commonly more numerous are nonphagocytizing histiocytes and less mature mononuclear cells characterized by a relatively large round to oval nucleus containing one or more nucleoli and surrounded by small to moderate amounts of basophilic cytoplasm (Figs. 5–1A and B). The latter cells simulate the large transformed lymphocyte and immunoblast.

The most important considerations in differential diagnosis are large cell or mixed large and small cell lymphoma, T-immuno-

blastic lymphoma, Hodgkin's disease, histiocytosis X, and pronounced benign reactive histiocytosis. The immunoperoxidase technique applied to standard marrow sections can be useful in verifying the identity of the histiocyte by demonstrating the presence of lysozyme, α_1-antitrypsin, or α_1-antichymotrypsin.[4, 6] Two other identifying enzyme ac-

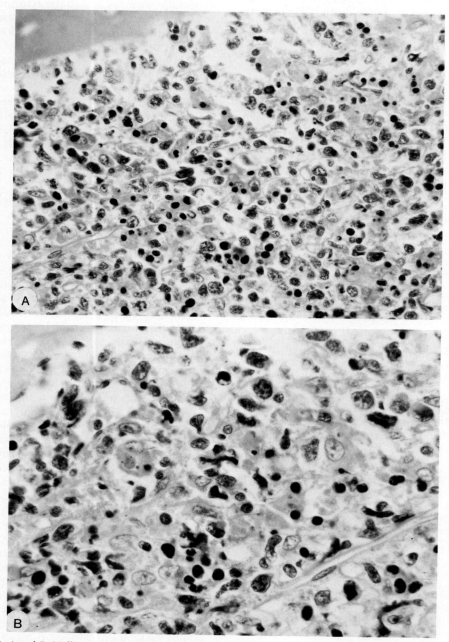

Figure 5–1. A and B. Malignant histiocytes at various stages of differentiation or maturation. The less differentiated histiocytes have large hyperchromatic nuclei and very little cytoplasm. The more differentiated have equally large but pale bland-appearing nuclei and abundant cytoplasm containing nucleated or more mature red cells. 400× and 680×, hematoxylin and eosin stain (H&E).

tivities, nonspecific esterase and acid phosphatase, are destroyed by the standard procedures applied to core marrow specimens. Demonstration of more than one immunoglobulin or light chain moiety in the cells is evidence against large cell and immunoblastic lymphoma, since histiocytes commonly phagocytize and thereby contain more than one of these proteins. In Hodgkin's disease, when many mononuclear variant cells are present, the presence of lymphocytes, Reed-Sternberg cells, varying degrees of fibroplasia, and the lack of phagocytosis generally clarify the diagnosis. In histiocytosis X the culprit cells are more uniform, have bland-appearing and folded nuclei, and are generally large by virtue of having more cytoplasm.

Development of malignant histiocytosis as a second neoplasm has been reported in treated cases of acute leukemia, most frequently in lymphoblastic leukemia of the T cell type.[7] Sufficient evidence has become available to contend that this is a profound reactive histiocytosis consequent to a viral infection occurring in immunologically suppressed patients rather than a second neoplasm.[8-10] The disease reported under various names, including familial erythrophagocytic lymphohistiocytosis, appears to be an exuberant histiocyte response to an overwhelming viral infection in the presence of an inborn error in histiocyte function.[11] In these pronounced reactive histiocytoses the marrow may be laden with mature histiocytes—mature by virtue of their abundant cytoplasm and small bland-appearing eccentrically placed nuclei. Phagocytosis, especially erythrophagocytosis, is usually strikingly apparent.

REFERENCES

1. Byrne, G. E., and Rappaport, H.: Malignant histiocytosis. *In* Akazaki, K., Rappaport, H., Berard, C. W., Bennett, J. M., and Ishikawa, E. (eds.): Malignant Diseases of the Hematopoietic System. Gann Monograph on Cancer Research 15. Tokyo, University of Tokyo Press, 1973, pp. 145–162.
2. Warnke, R. A., Kim, H., and Dorfman, R. F.: Malignant histiocytosis (histiocytosis medullary reticulosis). Cancer 35:215–230, 1975.
3. Vardiman, J. W., Byrne, G. E., and Rappaport, H.: Malignant histiocytosis with massive splenomegaly in asymptomatic patients. Cancer 36:419–427, 1975.
4. van der Valk, P., te Velde, J., Jansen, J., et al.: Malignant lymphoma of true histiocytic origin: Histiocytic sarcoma. Virchows Arch [Pathol Anat] 391:249–265, 1981.
5. Lampert, I. A., Catovsky, D., and Bergier, N.: Malignant histiocytosis: A clinico-pathologic study of 12 cases. Br J Haematol 40:65–77, 1978.
6. Mendelsohn, G., Eggleston, J. C., and Mann, R.: Relationship of lysozyme (muramidase) to histiocytic differentiation in malignant histiocytosis Cancer 45:273–279, 1980.
7. Starkie, C. M., Kenny, M. W., Mann, J. R., et al.: Histiocytic medullary reticulosis following acute lymphoblastic leukemia. Cancer 47:537–544, 1981.
8. Liu Yin, J. A., Kumaran, T. O., Marsh, G. W., et al.: Complete recovery of histiocytic medullary reticulosis-like syndrome in a child with acute lymphoblastic leukemia. Cancer 51:200–202, 1983.
9. Risdall, R. J., McKenna, R. W., Nesbit, M. E., et al.: Virus-associated hemophagocytic syndrome. Cancer 44:993–1002, 1979.
10. Jaffe, E. S., Costa, J., Fauci, A. S., et al.: Malignant lymphoma and erythrophagocytosis simulating malignant histiocytosis. Am J Med 75:741–749, 1983.
11. Perry, M. C., Harrison, E. G., Jr., Burgert, E. O., et al.: Familial erythrophagic lymphohistiocytosis. Cancer 38:209–218, 1976.

HISTIOCYTOSIS X (LANGERHANS' CELL HISTIOCYTOSIS)

Under the term histiocytosis X are grouped three apparently related diseases classically designated as *eosinophilic granuloma, Letterer-Siwe disease,* and *Hand-Schüller-Christian disease.*[1,2] Application of additional eponyms or of other terms such as differentiated histiocytosis, reticuloendotheliosis, or idiopathic inflammatory histiocytosis has served no etiologically clarifying or therapeutic purpose. More useful has been the dichotomy into localized and disseminated forms and the recognition of clinical and histological transitions between the three classic diseases. The basic character of the disease is as unsettled as its etiology. Current evidence favors neoplasia of the special form of histiocyte known as the Langerhans' cell rather than an unusual inflammatory or immunological response.[1] Thus, the associated immunological aberration manifested by a deficient function of suppressor T-lymphocytes in the disseminated form of the disease is probably consequent to, rather than the basis of, the histiocytosis. The eosinophilia, which is most evident in the more mature lesions and especially in eosinophilic granuloma, may be related to the elaboration of a chemotactic factor, possibly a prostaglandin, by the histiocytes. This would be analogous to the eosinophilia occurring in mast cell diseases.

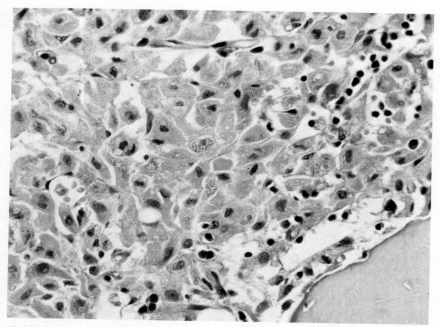

Figure 5–2. Epithelial-like histiocytic cells fill the marrow space in Letterer-Siwe disease. The cells are large, variable in shape consequent to pressing upon each other, and possess abundant nonvacuolated cytoplasm and a small bland nucleus that is frequently folded. 400×, H&E.

The disease commonly affects the skeleton at multiple sites, including the pelvis. Therefore, an iliac crest biopsy can be useful in providing histological evidence and thereby making unnecessary a formal surgical operation. This is particularly true in the disseminated form of the disease. Generalized marrow infiltration can be responsible for pancytopenia.

A variable histology in the marrow core

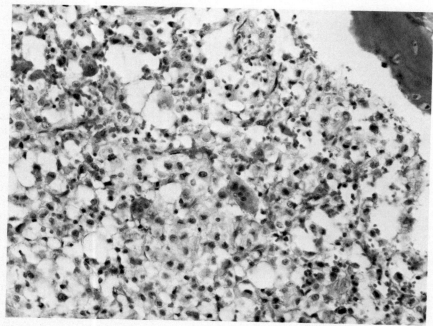

Figure 5–3. Heterogeneity characterizes the marrow lesion in eosinophilic granuloma in which the histiocytes may form multinucleated giant cells and are admixed with eosinophils and neutrophils. 250×, H&E.

specimen has been related to the stage of evolution of the lesions.[1,3] Younger lesions consist primarily of sheets of the histiocytes designated as HX cells, which are equivalent to Langerhans' cells, whereas older lesions contain variable numbers of eosinophils, lymphocytes, neutrophils, and pigment-laden histiocytes, commonly in association with necrotic foci. High lipid content of the histiocytes and formation of multinucleated giant cells are usually indicative of older lesions. These features can be related to the three classically recognized forms of histiocytosis X. In Letterer-Siwe disease the marrow contains clusters of bulky histiocytes with bland-appearing nuclei that commonly are folded. They are mixed with lesser numbers of eosinophils and lymphocytes (Fig. 5–2). Phagocytosis of red cells and granulocytes as well as hemosiderin deposition may be present. In Hand-Schüller-Christian disease foamy histiocytes are the predominant cell. Cytologically these cells may be indistinguishable from those occurring in hyperlipoproteinemia. In eosinophilic granuloma the mixtures of histiocytes and eosinophils are interspersed with varying numbers of prominent multinucleated giant cells (Fig. 5–3). Histological foci of each may closely resemble or be indistinguishable from the others. Trabecular bone destruction is commonly present.

REFERENCES

1. Nezelof, C.: Histiocytosis X: A histological and histogenetic study. *In* Rosenberg, H. S., and Bernstein, J. (eds.): Perspectives in Pediatric Pathology. Vol. 5. New York, Masson Publishing USA, Inc., 1979, pp. 153–178.
2. Rappaport, H.: Tumors of the hematopoietic system. Atlas of Tumor Pathology. Section 3. Fascicle 8. Washington, D. C., Armed Forces Institute of Pathology, 1966, pp. 63–91.
3. Nezelof, C., Frileux-Herbet, F., and Cronier-Sachot, J.: Disseminated histiocytosis X. Cancer 44: 1824–1838, 1979.

BENIGN REACTIVE HISTIOCYTOSIS

The occurrence of diffuse histiocytosis in the marrow as a benign reaction rather than as an inevitable malignant proliferation has gained special significance over the past decade. During this time successive reports asserted the development of histiocytic medullary reticulosis as a lethal complication of acute lymphoblastic leukemia.[1,2] This sequela always appeared within one year following diagnosis and successful chemotherapy of the leukemia. The association with acute myeloblastic or acute myelomonocytic leukemia has been reported less commonly.[3] Recently, this interpretation has been challenged by evidence that this histiocytosis is consequent to a virus infection, is self-limiting or remediable and reversible, and therefore is reactive rather than neoplastic.[4] An analogous conclusion has been proffered for a fatal complication developing in malignant lymphoma.[5] This view is supported by the recognition of a similar, if not identical, event occurring in patients immunosuppressed for renal transplantation.[6,7] The occurrence in patients without drug-induced immunosuppression, who have viral or bacterial infections, has also been noted.[6,8]

A similar disease has been observed in infants and young children, many of whom are siblings. An inherited immunological defect involving histiocyte function is a postulated basis.[9] *Familial erythrophagocytic lymphohistiocytosis* is one of several names applied to this disorder.

Clinically the features mimic those of histiocytic medullary reticulosis and consist of abrupt onset, fever, lymph node enlargement, and hepatomegaly or splenomegaly, or both. Peripheral blood cytopenias are the rule, but only rarely are circulating histiocytes detected.

The marrow is usually hypocellular, owing to a decrease in granulocyte and red cell precursors. Diagnostically there is a striking increase in histiocytes, which may be more obvious in smear preparations than in core specimen sections. The histiocytes exhibit all the characteristics of fully differentiated mature cells, and many are functioning macrophages with ingested red cells, platelets, and nucleated cells (Figs. 5–4 to 5–6). The histiocytosis is usually transient but may persist for several months.

The most critical differential consideration is histiocytic medullary reticulosis, perhaps better designated as malignant histiocytosis. In the final analysis, the distinction between benign and malignant histiocytosis depends on the morphology of the histiocytes, which are frankly benign with conspicuous macrophage function in reactive histiocytosis and frankly malignant with little if any phagocytosis in malignant histiocytosis. In the latter

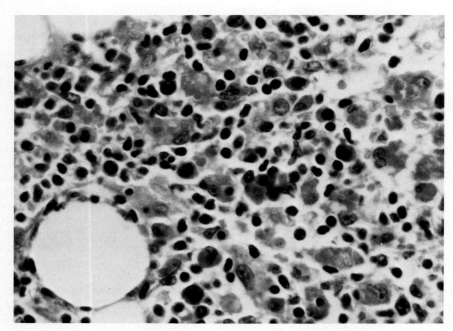

Figure 5–4. Serologically positive infectious mononucleosis complicated by jaundice, gluteal abscess, and purpura in a teen-age girl with moderately severe pancytopenia. The marrow contains numerous histiocytes, many of which show cytophagocytosis. Initially the diagnosis of histiocytic medullary reticulosis was considered. The patient recovered and is alive and well nine years later. 680×, H&E.

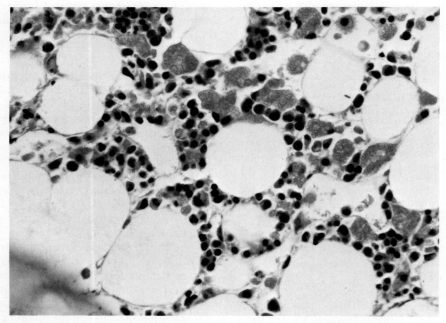

Figure 5–5. Mycosis fungoides that was present for about ten years in a middle-aged man treated with topical steroids, topical nitrogen mustard, and ultraviolet light. Development of generalized lymph node enlargement and splenomegaly suggested dissemination. The marrow contains many histiocytes showing intense erythrophagocytosis, but there is no mycosis fungoides. 400×, H&E.

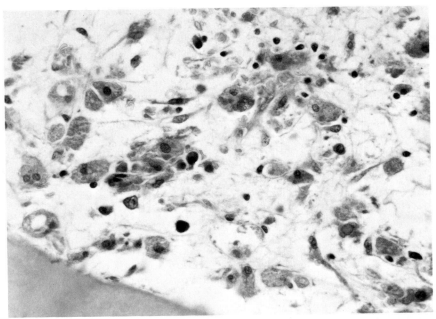

Figure 5–6. Undifferentiated small cell carcinoma of the lung in a middle-aged man who received chemotherapy. The hypocellular marrow contains numerous plump bland-appearing histiocytes with little evidence of cytophagocytosis. 400×, H&E.

condition marrow involvement may be far less obvious than in the former.

Lesser degrees of reactive histiocytosis with erythrophagocytosis occur in hemolytic anemia of various causes. In this context, the nidus of ingested red cells is usually more conspicuous than the phagocytizing histiocyte. Reactive histiocytosis rarely follows the cellular depletion phase in the chemotherapy of acute leukemia or in other cancers.

REFERENCES

1. Karcher, D. S., Head, D. R., and Mullins, J. D.: Malignant histiocytosis occurring in patients with acute lymphocytic leukemia. Cancer 41:1967–1973, 1978.
2. Starkie, C. M., Kenny, M. W., Mann, J. R., et al.: Histiocytic medullary reticulosis following acute lymphoblastic leukemia. Cancer 47:537–544, 1981.
3. Castoldi, G., Grusovin, G. D., Scapoli, G., et al.: Acute myelomonocytic leukemia terminating in histiocytic medullary reticulosis. Cancer 40:1735–1747, 1977.
4. Liu Yin, J. A., Kumaran, T. O., Marsh, G. W., et al.: Complete recovery of histiocytic medullary reticulosis-like syndrome in a child with acute lymphoblastic leukemia. Cancer 51:200–202, 1983.
5. Jaffe, E. S., Costa, J., Fauci, A. S., et al.: Malignant lymphoma and erythrophagocytosis simulating malignant histiocytosis. Am J Med 75:741–749, 1983.
6. Risdall, R. J., McKenna, R. W., Nesbit, M. E., et al.: Virus-associated hemophagocytic syndrome. Cancer 44:993–1002, 1979.
7. McKenna, R. W., Risdall, R. J., and Brunning, R. D.: Virus associated hemophagocytic syndrome. Hum Pathol 12:395–398, 1981.
8. Chandra, P., Chaudbery, S. A., Rosner, F., et al.: Transient histiocytosis with striking phagocytosis of platelets, leukocytes, and erythrocytes. Arch Intern Med 135:989–991, 1975.
9. Perry, M. C., Harrison, E. G., Jr., Burgert, E. O., et al.: Familial erythrophagocytic lymphohistiocytosis. Cancer 38:209–218, 1976.

LIPID STORAGE DISEASES (LIPID STORAGE HISTIOCYTOSES)

By virtue of containing macrophages, the marrow can be the site of perverse lipid accumulation either on a heritable or an acquired basis. Of the several heritable lipid storage diseases precisely defined by chemical, metabolic, and genetic analysis, in only two is bone marrow examination consistently useful diagnostically: *Gaucher's disease* and *Niemann-Pick's disease*. In both disorders a progressive macrophage proliferation occurs as a response to a specific hydrolytic enzyme deficiency, with a consequent accumulation in the macrophages of one or more metabolites of cell membrane lipids derived largely from red blood cells, leukocytes, and platelets.

Gaucher's disease, the most common of this group of unusual diseases, is caused by a deficient activity of glucocerebrosidase.[1] Ever increasing numbers of macrophages collect in the marrow, spleen, liver, and lymph nodes to store the glucocerebroside and produce the Gaucher's cell (Fig. 5–7). This cell is characterized by its large size (up to 100 μm in diameter), a small centrally to eccentrically placed nucleus, and abundant pale-staining cytoplasm with a texture likened to that of crumpled tissue paper. The cytoplasmic appearance is related to large numbers of elongated and distended lysosomes filled with the sphingolipid, which is arranged in stacks of slender tightly packed and twisted bilayers.[2] In hematoxylin-eosin–stained sections the cytoplasm of some Gaucher's cells is diffusely brown because of ferritin. When the section is treated with the PAS reagents the stored glucocerebroside reacts to produce a red to purplish-red Schiff complex. Pretreatment of the section with diastase does not abolish the reaction.

Progressive displacement of the normal hematopoietic cells in the marrow by Gaucher's cells together with increased splenic sequestration of circulating cells eventually results in peripheral blood cytopenias. There may be an increase in plasma cells in the marrow. Bone erosion may be severe and precipitate fracture. Rarely, there is necrosis of the marrow and bone.

Gaucher-like or pseudo-Gaucher's cells appear in the marrow in small numbers in several hematological diseases, including chronic granulocytic leukemia, acute myeloblastic leukemia, thalassemia, immune thrombocytopenia, and aplastic anemia.[3, 4] They are rarely detected in the lymphoproliferative diseases. Their presence probably reflects a rate of cell destruction in these diseases that exceeds the capacity of the marrow macrophages to metabolize the cerebrosides generated from membranes of phagocytized cells or cell fragments.[4] Subtle

ultrastructural differences between quasi- and authentic Gaucher's cells have been reported, but in standard sections they are hardly distinguishable.

Niemann-Pick's disease is metabolically analogous to Gaucher's disease and for like reasons induces macrophage proliferation for the storage of sphingomyelin because of a deficient activity of sphingomyelinase.[5] This impediment is probably also responsible for the coaccumulation of cholesterol, lysobisphosphatidic acid, and gangliosides in the macrophages.

The characteristic Niemann-Pick's cell is large (up to 90 μm in diameter), with a small eccentric nucleus and abundant pale-staining, finely vacuolated, or foamy cytoplasm (Fig. 5–8). In the hematoxylin-eosin–stained section some of the cells contain a yellow or yellowish brown pigment considered to be ceroid or its equivalent, lipofuscin. When the section is treated with Giemsa stain, some of the macrophages may have cytoplasmic blue or bluish green granules, which are the basis for the appellation *sea-blue histiocyte*.[6, 7]

The foamy, the ceroid, and the sea-blue types of macrophages are not specific for Niemann-Pick's disease. The significance of the latter two types has been a source of controversy. Both appear to owe their tinctorial properties to certain moieties or degradation products of complex lipids. All three types of macrophages have been identified in several of the well-characterized lipid storage diseases, including Wolman's disease, familial lipoprotein deficiency, familial hyperlipoproteinemia, lecithin-cholesterol acyltransferase deficiency, Fabry's disease, and some of the gangliosidoses (Figs. 5–9A and B).[7, 8] Some cases previously designated as primary sea-blue histiocytosis have proved to be adult nonneuronopathic Niemann-Pick's disease.[7, 9]

As in the case of the Gaucher's cell, small numbers of all of these macrophages can be found in the marrow in several of the primary hematological diseases, including acute myeloblastic leukemia, chronic granulocytic leukemia, polycythemia vera, erythroleukemia, thalassemia, sickle cell disease, and immune thrombocytopenia.[4, 7, 8] Again, this finding is considered a secondary response reflecting an accelerated cell destruction.[4] It may be concluded that the sea-blue and ceroid histiocytes are no more etiologically specific than the hemosiderin-laden macrophage.

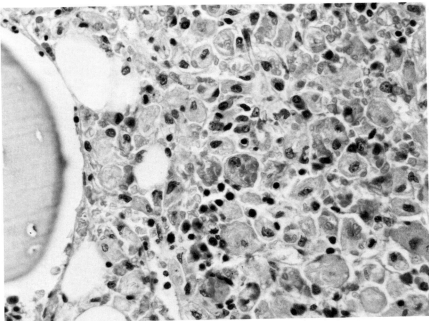

Figure 5–7. Gaucher's cells fill the intertrabecular space at the expense of the normal cell population. The Gaucher's cell is a large histiocyte with abundant wrinkled or creased-appearing cytoplasm and a small bland nucleus. 400×, H&E.

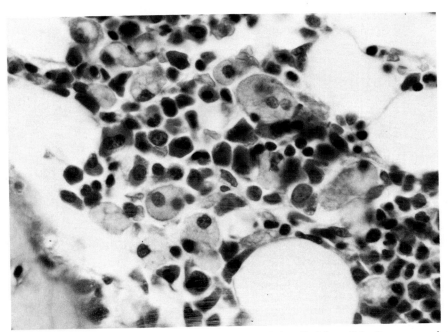

Figure 5–8. Niemann-Pick cells are mixed with normal hematopoietic cells. Most of the former are obviously larger than the developing blood cells and are characterized by irregularly vacuolated cytoplasm and a bland nucleus. 680×, H&E.

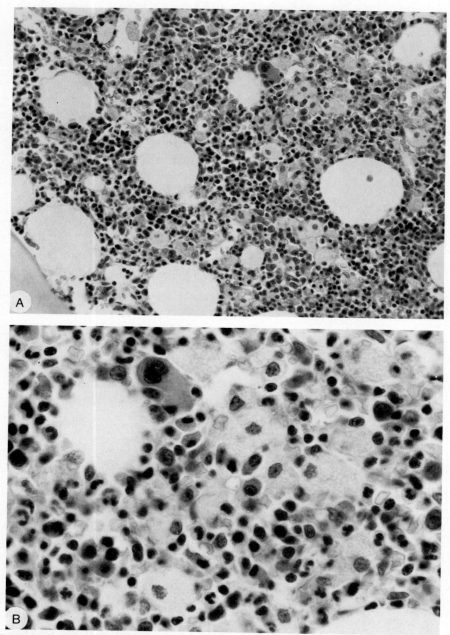

Figure 5–9. *A* and *B*. Foamy histiocytes in the marrow of a patient with hyperlipoproteinemia. The concentration of serum triglyceride was 1242 mg/dl, and that of cholesterol was 312 mg/dl. In smear preparations of aspirated marrow the cytoplasmic vacuoles of the foam cells failed to stain with the Wright-Giemsa stain but stained intensely with the Oil-Red-O dye, which confirmed the presence of neutral lipid. 250× and 680×, H&E.

REFERENCES

1. Brady, R. O., and Barranger, J. A.: Glucosylceramide lipidosis: Gaucher's disease. *In* Stanbury, J. B., Wyngaarden, J. B., Fredrickson, D. S., Goldstein, J. L., and Brown, M. S. (eds.): The Metabolic Basis of Inherited Diseases. 5th ed. New York, McGraw-Hill, 1983, pp. 842–856.
2. Lee, R. W., Peters, S. P., and Glew, R. H.: Gaucher's disease: Clinical, morphologic, and pathogenetic considerations. *In* Sommers, J. C., and Rosen, P. P. (eds.): Pathology Annual. Part 2. New York, Appleton-Century-Crofts, 1977, pp. 309–339.
3. Dosek, H., Rosner, F., and Sawitzky, A.: Acquired lipidosis: Gaucher-like cells and "blue cells" in chronic granulocytic leukemia. Semin Hematol 9:309–316, 1972.
4. Haykoe, F. G. J., Flemans, R. J., and Cowling, D. C.: Acquired lipidosis of marrow macrophages. J Clin Pathol 32:420–428, 1979.
5. Brady, R. O.: Sphingomyelin lipidosis: Niemann-Pick's disease. *In* Stanbury, J. G., Wyngaarden, J. B., Fredrickson, D. S., Goldstein, J. L., and Brown, M. S. (eds.): The Metabolic Basis of Inherited Diseases. 5th ed. New York, McGraw-Hill, 1983, pp. 831–841.
6. Rywlin, A. M., Hernandez, J. A., Chastain, D. E., et al.: Ceroid histiocytosis of spleen and bone marrow in idiopathic thrombocytopenic purpura (ITP): A contribution to the understanding of the sea-blue histiocyte. Blood 37:587–593, 1971.
7. Dawson, P. J., and Dawson, G.: Adult Niemann-Pick disease with sea-blue histiocytes in the spleen. Hum Pathol 13:1115–1120, 1982.
8. Tachibana, F., Hakozaki, H., Takahashi, K., et al.: Syndrome of the sea-blue histiocyte. Acta Pathol Jpn 29:73–97, 1979.
9. Quattrin, N.: Sea blue histiocytosis. *In* Seno, S., Takaku, F., and Irino, S. (eds.): The Proceedings of the 16th International Congress of Hematology. Amsterdam, Excerpta Medica, 1977, pp. 1018–1043.

GRANULOMAS

Reduced to its minimum, the granuloma consists of a cluster of macrophages, some or all of which may have evolved to epithelioid cells (Fig. 5–10).[1] The addition of features such as giant cells and necrosis produce a more complex granuloma, but these accessories are of limited value as etiological clues, since there are documented exceptions to every rule relating histology to causes of granulomas. Whether giant cells are of the foreign body or Langhans' type, whether necrosis is present or not, and whether there are lymphocytes, plasma cells, neutrophils, or eosinophils surrounding the granuloma are not etiologically determinative in any given case (Figs. 5–11 to 5–13). Microorganisms must be sought by using special histological stains, and culture must be done in all cases. The single exception to this caveat is the lipogranuloma in its early formative stage. Prior to the development of epithelioid cells or giant cells, this lesion consists of a poorly circumscribed cluster of macrophages con-

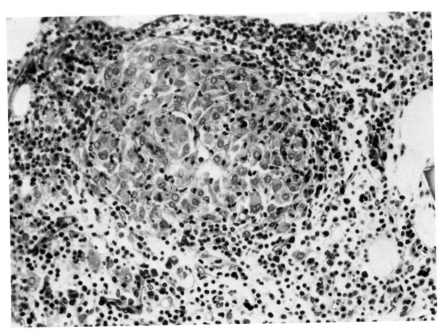

Figure 5–10. Granuloma consisting principally of epithelioid cells in a case of atypical mycobacterial infection. 250×, H&E.

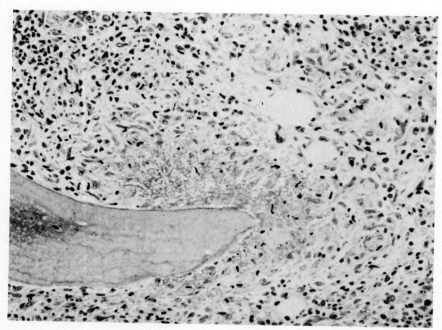

Figure 5–11. Necrotizing granuloma centered around a trabecula in a case of tuberculosis complicating acute myeloblastic leukemia after chemotherarpy. 250×, H&E.

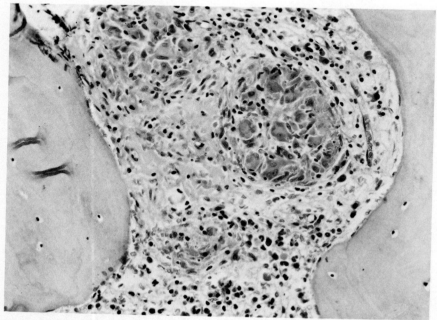

Figure 5–12. Granulomas complete with multinucleated giant cells almost surrounded by a ring of collagen fibrosis in a case of sarcoidosis. 250×, H&E.

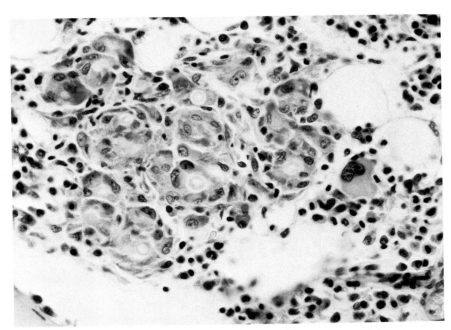

Figure 5–13. Clusters of macrophages converting into epithelioid and multinucleated giant cells and engulfing cryptococcus organisms. 400×, H&E.

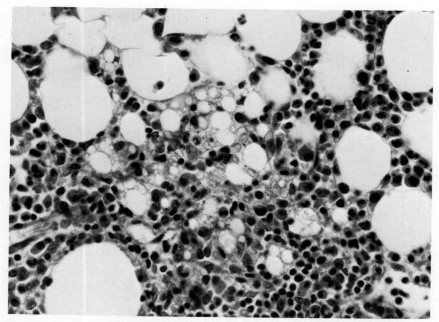

Figure 5–14. Lipogranuloma in an early formative stage is composed of poorly circumscribed histiocytes with clusters of round to oval optically empty vacuoles of varying size that are mingled with marrow cells. 400×, H&E.

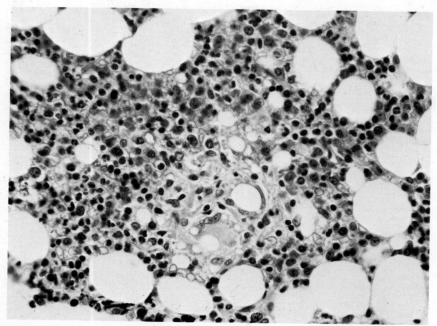

Figure 5–15. Lipogranuloma in a more advanced stage of development contains vacuolated multinucleated giant cells. The assortment of vacuoles of varying size is typical of the lipogranuloma. 400×, H&E.

taining or surrounding small lipid droplets, allegedly of mineral oil or oily radiographic contrast medium (Figs. 5–14 to 5–16A and B). Later in their evolution, the lipogranulomas cannot be decisively distinguished from granulomas of a more serious nature.[2, 3]

Granulomas in the marrow indicate either a systemic disease that has spread by hematogenous dissemination or a local reaction to the deposition of an inanimate foreign substance. The putative causes of the granulomatous response are numerous.[4, 5] Fortu-

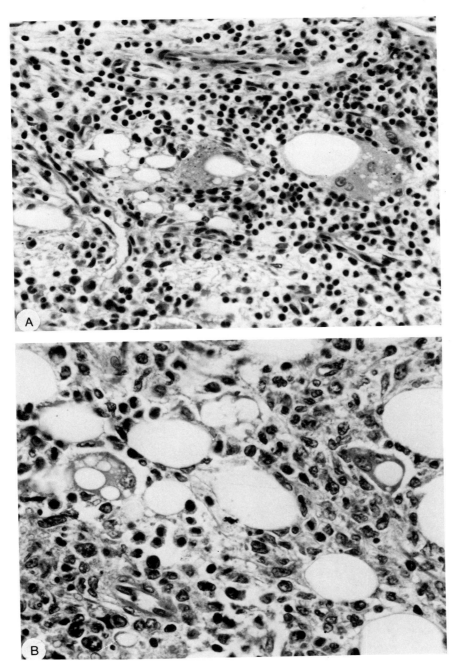

Figure 5–16. *A* and *B*. Lipogranuloma with vacuolated giant cells. This picture is well known to occur in lymphodes after lymphangiography with an oily contrast medium. 400× and 520×, H&E.

nately, causes proved or invoked for marrow granulomas are relatively few. The common causes and associations are listed in Table 5–1.

Table 5–1. Granulomas: Etiologies and Associations

I. Infectious
    Tuberculosis*
    Atypical mycobacterial infection*
    Fungus infection, especially histoplasmosis*
    Brucellosis
    Infectious mononucleosis
    Viral hepatitis
    Typhoid
    Leprosy
II. Sarcoidosis*
III. Malignant tumors
    Hodgkin's disease*
    Non-Hodgkin's lymphoma
      Poorly differentiated lymphocytic lymphoma
      Large cell lymphoma
      Immunoblastic lymphoma
IV. Renal osteodystrophy*
V. Drug hypersensitivity

---

*Most frequent in the marrow of a general hospital population.

In the search for granulomas in the marrow, the core marrow specimen is superior to smear preparations of marrow particles and may have some advantage over sections of aspirated particles. Aspiration may disrupt granulomas and thus obscure their morphology, and fibrosis surrounding some granulomas may prevent their aspiration (Fig. 5–12).

REFERENCES

1. Adams, D. O.: The granulomatous inflammatory response. Am J Pathol 84:164–191, 1976.
2. Rywlin, A. M., and Ortega, R.: Lipid granulomas of the bone marrow. Am J Clin Pathol 57:457–462, 1972.
3. Pak, H. Y., and Friedman, N. B.: Pseudosarcoid granulomas in Hodgkin's disease. Hum Pathol 12:832–837, 1981.
4. Pease, G. L.: Granulomatous lesions in bone marrow. Blood 11:720–734, 1956.
5. Ellman, L.: Bone marrow biopsy in the evaluation of lymphoma, carcinoma and granulomatous disorders. Am J Med 60:1–7, 1976.

MAST CELL PROLIFERATIVE DISEASES

CONCEPT AND SCOPE

Of the cellular inhabitants of the marrow, the mast cell appears to be the least numerous, the least conspicuous, and the least common perpetrator of proliferative diseases. Evidence from several sources suggests that the mast cell stems from the monocyte and thus is a distant relative of the granulocyte.[1] Like the basophil, from which it is morphologically and cytogenetically distinct, the mast cell contains a long list of complex compounds and factors to which are ascribed almost as many functions.[2] All of these are of interest, but few can be related to significant marrow pathology. The functions that may have a role are (1) the eosinophilic chemotactic factor, which may explain the frequent marrow and blood eosinophilia associated with mast cell diseases,[2, 3] (2) heparin and prostaglandins, both of which may be directly or indirectly responsible for the osseous lesions,[3, 4] and (3) factors promoting wound healing, which may provoke the perivascular and paratrebecular fibrosis.[3]

Under normal circumstances, mast cells in the standard marrow core section are easily overlooked, although they tend to congregate adjacent to blood vessels. Morphologically they differ from all other cells by virtue of the unique combination of a large size, a round nucleus, and a cytoplasm filled with metachromatic granules. Unfortunately, the contents of the granules are relatively unstable, so that this insignia is largely lost in the standard preparation of the marrow core

section. In properly stained marrow smear preparations or in specially prepared sections, however, the metachromatic granules remain intact, and the mast cells are readily detected.[5]

Only two diseases of mast cells involving the marrow are sufficiently characterized to deserve treatment here: systemic mast cell disease and the eosinophilic fibrohistiocytic lesion. These may, in fact, be different stages or aspects of the same disease.[6]

Reactive mast cell hyperplasia occurs in few diseases and usually to an inconspicuous degree. These diseases are generalized or selective medullary aplasia, senescent osteoporosis, and the lymphoproliferative diseases.[7]

REFERENCES

1. Lennert, K., and Parwaresch, M. R.: Mast cells and mast cell neoplasia: A review. Histopathology 3:349–365, 1979.
2. Metcalfe, D. D., and Kaliner, M.: Mast cells and basophils. *In* Oppenheim, J. J., Rosenstreich, D. L., and Potter, M. (eds.): Cellular Functions in Immunity and Inflammation. New York, Elsevier/North Holland, 1981, pp. 301–322.
3. Cryer, P. E., and Kissane, J. M. (eds.): Clinicopathologic Conference: Systemic mastocytosis. Am J Med 61:671–680, 1976.
4. Cryer, P. E., and Kissane, J. M. (eds.): Clinicopathologic Conference: Osteopenia. Am J Med 69:915–922, 1980.
5. te Velde, J., Vismans, F. J. F. E., Leenheers-Binnendijk, L., et al.: The eosinophilic fibrohistiocytic lesion of the bone marrow. Virchows Arch [Pathol Anat] 377:277–285, 1978.
6. Fallon, M. D., Whyte, M. P., and Teitelbaum, S. T.:

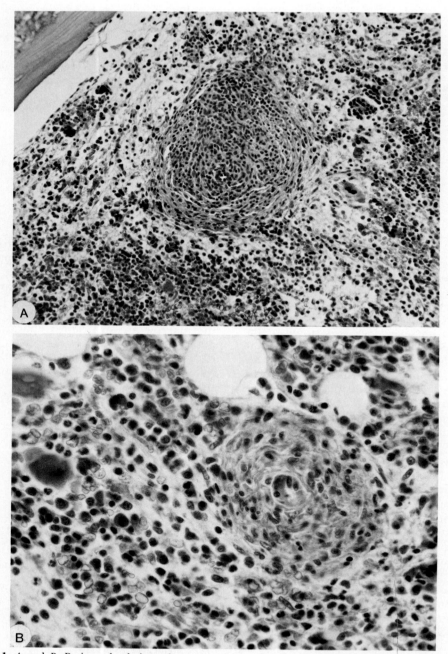

Figure 6–1. *A* and *B*. Perivascular lesions characterized by concentric rings of collagen studded with mast cells enclosing a small artery. 170× and 400×, hematoxylin and eosin stain (H&E).

Systemic mastocytosis associated with generalized osteopenia. Hum Pathol 12:813–820, 1981.

7. Webb, T. A., Li, C. Y., and Yam, L. T.: Systemic mast cell disease. A clinical and hematopathologic study of 26 cases. Cancer 49:927–938, 1982.

SYSTEMIC MAST CELL DISEASE

This disease is among the least common of the diseases that can be classified as primary hematopoietic diseases. Many of its clinical manifestations, including urticaria, flushing, diarrhea, and osteoporosis are attributed to the histamine, heparin, and other compounds elaborated by the mast cells.[1–3]

Systemic mast cell disease, whether benign or malignant, involves the marrow.[1–3] Since the pelvic bones are a frequently affected skeletal site, the standard core biopsy specimen can be diagnostic. Most cases show a focal perivascular or paratrabecular aggregation of mast cells associated with a remarkable form of collagen fibrosis (Figs. 6–1A and B, 6–2).[1, 3, 4] This telltale fibrosis is structured in lamellated layers or rings that abut against bone trabecula or form shells around small blood vessels. The mast cells are insinuated between the collagen lamellae and in the standard marrow section are undistinguished cells with round to elongated nuclei. A less

structured, patchy fibrosis may also be present, and small clusters of mast cells may be scattered through the remaining marrow. Granulocytic hyperplasia is usually present with an increase in eosinophils, which may be reflected in the blood.[5] Only rarely is there diffuse mast cell infiltration that is analogous to an acute myeloblastic leukemia. Excepting these latter cases, distinguishing a benign from a malignant mast cell proliferation, that is, a hyperplasia from a leukemia, may not be feasible solely from the morphology. Attempts have been made to resolve this problem by using cytochemistry.[1]

In the majority of cases osteoporosis or osteosclerosis, or both, is present.[2] This condition is most intense in the vertebrae and may not be evident in the iliac crest biopsy specimen.

Progression of benign to malignant forms of mast cell disease has been reported, as has the development of myeloid and monocytic leukemia.[1]

A relation between the eosinophilic fibrohistiocytic (mastocellular) lesion and marrow mastocytosis is difficult to establish.[6] Both are manifested by localized mastocytosis, fibrosis, and perivascular localization, and both are associated with osteoporosis, especially of the vertebrae. Some of the cases recorded as

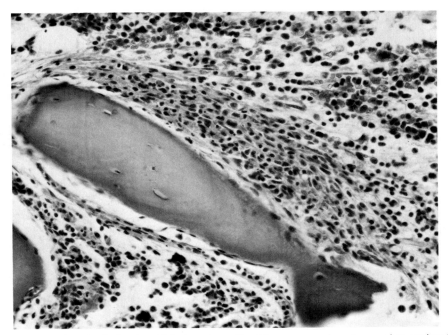

Figure 6–2. A paratrabecular lesion in which the mast cells with accompanying stroma abut against bone. 250×, H&E.

systemic mastocytosis may in fact be the eo-sinophilic fibrohistiocytic (mastocellular) le-sion, or the latter condition may be an incip-ient form of systemic mastocytosis.

REFERENCES

1. Lennert, K., and Parwaresch, M. R.: Mast cells and mast cell neoplasia: A review. Histopathology 3:349–365, 1979.
2. Cryer, P. E., and Kissane, J. M. (eds.): Clinicopath-ologic Conference: Systemic mastocytosis. Am J Med 61:671–680, 1976.
3. Webb, T. A., Li, C. Y., and Yam, L. T.: Systemic mast cell disease. A clinical and hematopathologic study of 26 cases. Cancer 49:927–938, 1982.
4. Udoji, W. C., and Razavi, S. A.: Mast cells and myelofibrosis. Am J Clin Pathol 63:203–209, 1975.
5. Yam, L. T., Yam, C. F., and Li, C. Y.: Eosinophilia in systemic mastocytosis. Am J Clin Pathol 73:48–54, 1980.
6. te Velde, J., Vismans, F. J. F. E., Leenheers-Binnen-dijk, L., et al.: The eosinophilic fibrohistiocytic lesion of the bone marrow. Virchows Arch [Pathol Anat] 377:277–285, 1978.

EOSINOPHILIC FIBROHISTIOCYTIC (MASTOCELLULAR) LESION

An unusual lesion apparently limited to the bone marrow, the *eosinophilic fibrohistiocytic lesion,* was described in 1972 and ascribed to drug hypersensitivity.[1] A subsequent study revealed that the cells that originally were considered to be histiocytes converting into fibroblasts and designated as fibrohistiocytes are in fact mast cells.[2] In addition, the later study disclosed that all cases had vertebral osteoporosis, and most had vertebral frac-tures. The previously correlated drug hyper-sensitivity was not confirmed. Currently, the significance of the lesion appears to be three-fold: it is indicative of bone disease, it may be related to systemic mast cell disease from which distinction may not always be possible,[3] and it can be mistaken for Hodgkin's disease or angioimmunoblastic lymphadenopathy in the marrow.[4]

The lesions are focal, up to 2 mm in diameter, and are located around arterioles, sinusoids, and within or around lymphocyte aggregates (Figs. 6–3 to 6–5). The constituent cells are principally eosinophils and mast cells with lesser numbers of plasma cells and lym-phocytes. The mast cells are recognized by an elongated shape, oval to spindle-shaped nuclei, and amphophilic cytoplasm. The met-achromatic granules are poorly demon-strated or invisible in marrow core specimens processed by the standard method. The same is true for the Charcot-Leyden crystals pres-ent in most cases. Since the elongated mast cells simulate fibroblasts, the lesions have a

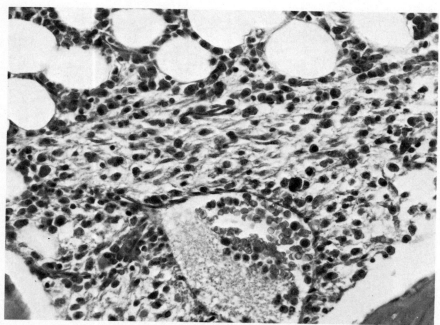

Figure 6–3. A perisinusoidal lesion in which mast cells admixed with eosinophils, lymphocytes, and plasma cells lie in a fibrillar stroma partially or completely surrounding a sinusoid. 325×, H&E.

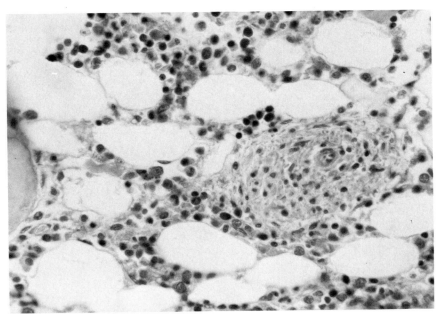

Figure 6–4. A periarteriolar lesion in which a thick ring of collagen containing mast cells coats a small vessel. Remarkably similar lesions occur in mast cell disease. 400×, H&E.

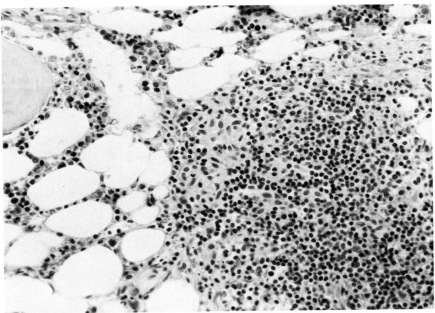

Figure 6–5. A lymphofollicular lesion in which a layer of mast cells surrounds an aggregate of well-differentiated lymphocytes. 250×, H&E.

fibroblastic appearance, but there may be no collagen and little if any increase in reticulin in some of the lesions. A striking eosinophilia and an increase in the number of mast cells is evident in the rest of the marrow.

In marrow core specimens obtained from the iliac crest there is little if any of the osteoporosis that is present in the vertebrae.

REFERENCES

1. Rywlin, A. M., Hoffman, E. P., and Ortega, R. S.: Eosinophilic fibrohistiocytic lesion of bone marrow. A distinctive new morphologic finding, probably related to drug hypersensitivity. Blood 40:464–472, 1972.

2. te Velde, J., Vismans, F. J. F. E., Leenheers-Binnendijk, L., et al.: The eosinophilic fibrohistiocytic lesion of the bone marrow. A mastocellular lesion in bone disease. Virchows Arch [Pathol Anat] 377:277–285, 1978.

3. Cryer, P. E., and Kissane, J. M., (eds.): Clinicopathologic Conference: Osteopenia. Am J Med 69:915–922, 1980.

4. Pangalis, G. A., Moran, E. M., and Rappaport, H.: Blood and bone marrow findings in angioimmunoblastic lymphadenopathy. Blood 51:71–83, 1978.

7

CYTOPENIAS NOT RELATED TO HEMATOPOIETIC MALIGNANCY

CONCEPT AND SCOPE

The search for the etiologies of most cytopenias that are manifested in the peripheral blood requires marrow examination. This rule is valid whether or not hematopoietic malignancy is being considered as a probable diagnosis. The exceptions to this principle are usually obvious, a case in point being characteristic nutritional iron deficiency in pediatric patients.

The marrow core specimen is especially useful in the diagnostic evaluation of these cases because quantification of the total hematopoietic population and of each cell lineage is more precise and reliable than are judgments based solely on smear preparations.

Cytopenias associated with a normal cellular attrition rate are as a rule more serious than those in which there is an accelerated loss, whether the loss is external as in gastrointestinal bleeding or internal as in accelerated splenic destruction. Clues to the state of marrow function may be present in the peripheral blood, such as the reticulocyte concentration, but these signs usually are more valuable for assessing the progress of a disease or the effect of therapy after the status of the marrow has been determined. Thus, in this group of diseases marrow core biopsy is considered optional or necessary only to exclude a diagnosis of a particular disease in cases of accelerated erythrolysis, granulocytolysis, or thrombocytolysis but is mandatory to establish a diagnosis of selective or generalized medullary hypoplasia or aplasia.

ANEMIA

Proper and complete evaluation of anemia requires examination of the marrow. There are obvious exceptions to this caveat, as exemplified by unequivocal cases caused by dietary iron deficiency in children. The multiplicity of causes and mechanisms of anemia requires that a planned diagnostic program be followed, and algorithms for this have been developed.[1,2] One traditional approach is to study the peripheral blood and to segregate cases on the basis of red cell size, chromaticity, and other morphological characteristics.

Analysis of the marrow core specimen in the study of anemia begins with the semi-quantification of marrow cellularity followed by an estimation of the abundance of nucleated red cells. Customarily, this estimation is related to the abundance of granulocytes and is stated in terms of a myeloid-erythroid ratio. The prevailing stage of red cell maturation is then assessed. As a rule, normoblastic maturation is manifested by a predominance of orthochromatic forms and megaloblastic maturation by a large majority of erythroblastic and basophilic forms. The amount of hemosiderin iron is graded. Finally, the status of the granulocyte and megakaryocyte series is evaluated.

Normoblastic Erythroid Hyperplasia. Marrow cellularity is usually increased, in some cases markedly. Characteristically, orthochromatic and polychromatophilic normoblasts prevail, and less mature forms are scarce or absent (Fig. 7–1). Granulocytes and megakaryocytes as a rule are unremarkable

121

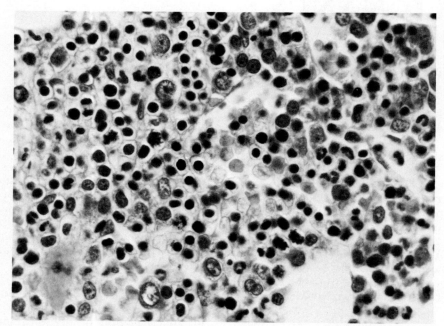

Figure 7–1. Normoblastic erythroid hyperplasia in which late-stage normoblasts, that is, orthochromatic and polychromatic forms, are more numerous than early-stage precursors, that is, basophilic normoblasts and erythroblasts. As the normoblast matures, its nucleus becomes smaller and denser. 680×, (H&E).

or somewhat increased. The amount of hemosiderin present is variable and depends on the cause, mechanism, and prior treatment of the anemia. In chronic hemolysis without hemosiderinuria, the amount of hemosiderin is commonly increased, sometimes to a striking degree, as in major thalassemias. On the other hand, in chronic bleeding iron stores may be depleted. In erythrocytosis—whether compensatory to hypoxia, stimulated by inappropriate erythropoietin secretion, or related to stress—the amount of hemosiderin is usually normal. The distinction between hyperplasia and polycythemia vera on the basis of the core specimen may not be possible in some cases, since iron stores can be depleted in both conditions.

Megaloblastic Erythroid Hyperplasia. The megaloblastosis resulting from vitamin B_{12} or folate deficiency produces a hyperplasia of the marrow, which usually packs the intertrabecular space completely. Strikingly prominent erythroblasts predominate to a degree that does not occur in normoblastic maturation (Fig. 7–2). Progress of maturation to the orthochromatic level is variable but usually limited. In some cases basophilic forms are especially common. This may be related to a concomitant iron deficiency. Orthochromatic megaloblasts can sometimes be identified, but usually the distinction between megaloblasts and normoblasts cannot be made with confidence on the basis of the core section.

In the granulocyte series giant metamyelocytes and band forms are more readily identified than hypersegmented neutrophils because in the latter all nuclear lobes rarely lie in the same plane of section (Figs. 7–2A and B). Megakaryocytes may be normal, slightly increased, or decreased in number. Frequently their morphology is remarkable for hyperlobation and lobular crowding of the nucleus to the periphery of the cell (Figs. 7–2B and C). Mitoses in all three series—erythroid, granulocytic, and megakaryocytic—are more numerous than normally. This situation reflects the protracted cell cycle and not an increased rate of cell division.

In at least half of the cases there are one or more aggregates of well-differentiated lymphocytes and many pericapillary plasma cells. These features have been linked to an immune factor in the pathogenesis of the megaloblastosis of pernicious anemia. The amount of hemosiderin may be normal, decreased, or overly abundant.

The distinction between megaloblastic proliferation and erythroleukemia may be difficult to make in the core biopsy section unless the granulocytic and megakaryocytic abnormalities can be recognized. This differentiation is more reliably based on the assays of vitamin B_{12} and folate metabolism used in establishing the etiology of the megaloblastosis.

Hemosiderin. The amount of iron present as hemosiderin can be evaluated in a hematoxylin-eosin–stained section prepared from suitably processed core specimens. Overexposure to demineralizing reagents must be avoided. Only hemosiderin contained within macrophages is considered to represent authentic storage iron. Ferritin, although a proper component of iron stores, is not considered because it is not visualized by light microscopy. The Prussian blue stain can be used to confirm that the pigment is hemosiderin. There is a consensus that morphological examination of the marrow for hemosiderin is the most reliable and economical method currently available to assess body iron stores. Some studies indicate that the core section is more precise than the particle smear in this evaluation.[3, 4] Estimation of the amount of hemosiderin present in sections can be conveniently graded according to the scale proposed by Krause: Grade 0 = no hemosiderin; Grade I = fine granules in every 3 to 4 high-power fields (hpf); Grade II = heavy granules in every 2 to 3 hpf; Grade III = a few granules in every hpf; and Grade IV = larger amounts.[4]

Lack of iron occurs in a wide variety of chronic diseases as well as in the common circumstances of inadequate dietary intake and chronic bleeding. Depletion of iron is almost characteristic of polycythemia vera, in contrast to the adequate amounts in compensatory and spurious erythrocytoses. On the other hand, a surfeit of hemosiderin iron is most commonly related to a lack of utilization, as in medullary aplasia and leukemia, to an excessive intake primarily consequent to multiple transfusions, as in major thalassemias and refractory anemias, or to an apparently impaired release of iron from macrophages, as in the anemias of many chronic diseases.

By this stage in the analysis of most cases of anemia obvious features or subtle clues have been recognized that provide a definite diagnosis or a circumscribed number of diagnostic possibilities. Most commonly in cases subjected to biopsy the diagnosis is one of the following: (1) aplastic or hypoplastic ane-

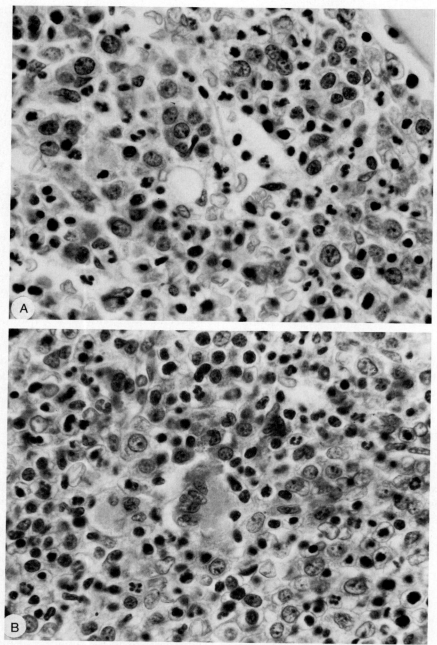

Figure 7–2. *A, B,* and *C.* Megaloblastic erythroid hyperplasia in which large early precursor cells are as abundant as or more abundant than small late precursors. This deviant proportioning, coupled with giant metamyelocytes, giant bands, hypersegmented granulocytes, and abnormal megakaryocytes, provides the morphological basis for the provisional diagnosis of this maturation defect. 680×, 680×, and 680×, H&E.

Illustration continued on opposite page

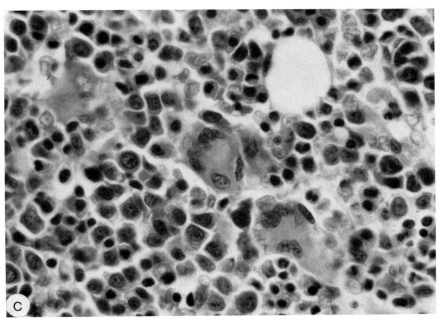

Figure 7–2. *Continued.*

mia; (2) leukemia or lymphoma; (3) metastatic cancer; (4) anemia of chronic disease with plasmacytosis, lymphocytosis, or renal osteodystrophy; (5) megaloblastic erythroid hyperplasia due to vitamin B_{12} or folate deficiency or to folate antimetabolites; (6) normoblastic erythroid hyperplasia related to chronic bleeding, chronic hemolysis, or dietary iron deficiency; and (7) refractory anemia with or without sideroblastosis or erythrodysplasia, that is, myelodysplasia. Specific features useful in the diagnosis of these diseases are described in the appropriate sections.

REFERENCES

1. Wintrobe, M. M., Lee, G. R., Boggs, D. R., Bithell, T. C., Foerster, J., Athens, J. W., and Lukers, J. N.: The approach to the patient with anemia. *In* Clinical Hematology. Chap. 20. Philadelphia, Lea & Febiger, 1981, pp. 529–558.
2. Hillman, R. S., and Finch, C. A.: Red Cell Manual. Philadelphia, F. A. Davis Company, 1974, pp. 23–51.
3. Ellis, L. D., Jensen, W. N., and Westerman, M. P.: Marrow iron. Ann Intern Med 61:44–49, 1964.
4. Krause, J. R., Brubaker, D. O., and Kaplan, J.: Comparison of stainable iron in aspirated and needle biopsy specimens of bone marrow. Am J Clin Pathol 72:68–70, 1979.

IMMUNE THROMBOCYTOPENIC PURPURA

The principal value of the marrow biopsy in this disease is to confirm the diagnoses by uncovering no other morphological basis for the thrombocytopenia. Etiological considerations of thrombocytopenia proceed most readily from quantification of megakaryocytes, with semiquantification being sufficient for clinical purposes. For this the core biopsy section is far more reliable than the aspirated and smeared preparation.

The normal marrow as represented in a standard histological section prepared from the iliac crest core specimen contains 12 to 25 megakaryocytes per sq mm.[1, 2] The cells almost always exist as singlets, randomly dispersed. Typically they are round to oval, contain abundant cytoplasm, and have four or more nuclear lobes in the plane of the section.

Irrespective of etiology, immune thrombocytopenia is always associated with a normal or an increased number of megakaryocytes. Megakaryocytosis is more commonly evident in chronic than in acute cases. In the chronic state the increase is considered to represent a compensatory hyperplasia. A

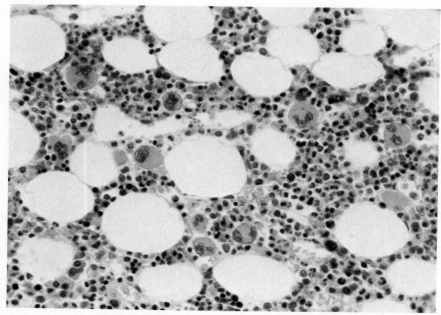

Figure 7–3. Acute thrombocytopenic purpura with a high titre of antiplatelet antibodies in an elderly man who was being treated with methyldopa and hydrochlorothiazide for systemic arterial hypertension. There is a moderately increased number of megakaryocytes, most of which are morphologically normal. 325×, H&E.

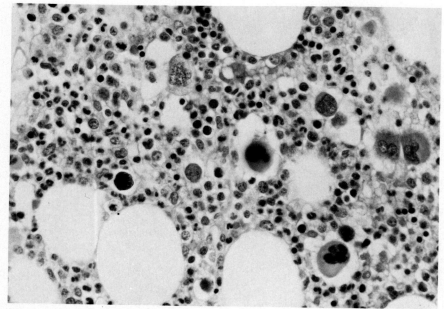

Figure 7–4. Chronic thrombocytopenia with a high titre of antiplatelet antibodies in an elderly man without acknowledged drug exposure. A moderately increased number of megakaryocytes is associated with a deficiency of cytoplasm in some of the megakaryocytes. 400×, H&E.

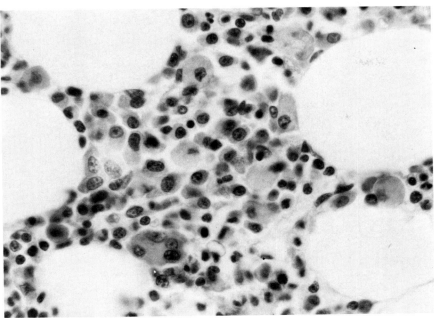

Figure 7–5. Chronic idiopathic thrombocytopenic purpura in which the marrow contains several groups of large mononuclear macrophages laden with brown cytoplasmic pigment. The macrophages are smaller than the single megakaryocyte represented. They should not be confused with micromegakaryocytes. 680×, H&E.

concentration of 35 to 40 per sq mm or greater can be accepted with assurance as elevated.[1,2] Qualitative changes are not as reliable an indicator of this disorder as is quantification. There may be an increase of megakaryocytes devoid of cytoplasm or of immature megakaryocytes characterized by hypolobulated nuclei and small amounts of basophilic cytoplasm (Figs. 7–3 and 7–4). This morphology in conjunction with the detection of antiplatelet antibodies in the serum or bound to platelets establishes the diagnosis in both acute and chronic cases in children and adults.[3,4] In an occasional instance there are groups of enlarged histiocytes containing pigment (Fig. 7–5).[5] Their genesis is probably analogous to that of the pseudo-Gaucher's cells formed in the marrow in chronic granulocytic leukemia.

Normoblastic erythroid hyperplasia may be present consequent to bleeding or less commonly to coexisting hemolytic anemia (Evans' syndrome). Only hyaline thrombi in the marrow blood vessels serve to distinguish this morphology from that of thrombotic thrombocytopenic purpura or disseminated intravascular coagulation (Fig. 7–6).

In the differential diagnostic considerations of thrombocytopenia, amegakaryocytic or hypomegakaryocytic thrombocytopenia is readily identified in the core biopsy specimen. Use of the aspirated and smeared preparation for this diagnosis is unreliable. The causes of a scarcity or absence of megakaryocytes are numerous and include generalized medullary aplasia, leukemia and lymphoma as the most frequent.

Thrombocytopenia with compensatory megakaryocytosis is rarely confused with a leukemia in which there can be an increase in megakaryocytes. Increases are common in chronic granulocytic leukemia and polycythemia vera, but associated abnormalities in the granulocytes and normoblasts, respectively, are predominant. In essential thrombocythemia, the megakaryocytes occur in large cohesive groups, whereas in chronic primary myelofibrosis at least some of the numerous and bizarre megakaryocytes are entrapped in collagen. Large numbers of micromegakaryocytes are typical of the megakaryocytic phase of chronic granulocytic leukemia. Finally, in acute megakaryocytic leukemia many atypical megakaryocytes are admixed with myeloblasts and erythroblasts in a coarse reticulin network.

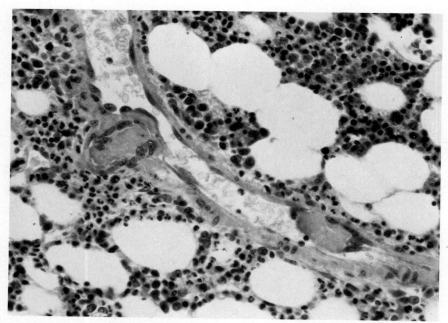

Figure 7–6. Acute disseminated intravascular coagulation manifested by purpura, severe thrombocytopenia, decreased plasma fibrinogen levels, and increased fibrin split products and fibrin monomer concentrations in the blood of a man who had cardiac valve replacement surgery. Small vessel thrombi were detected in the marrow, skin, and lungs. 325×, H&E.

REFERENCES

1. Ellis, J. T., and Peterson, P.: The bone marrow in polycythemia vera. *In* Sommers, J. C. (ed.): Pathology Annual. Vol. 14. Part 1. New York, Appleton-Century-Crofts, 1979, pp. 383–403.
2. Branehög, I., Kutti, J., Ridell, B., et al.: The relation of thrombokinetics to bone marrow megakaryocytes in idiopathic thrombocytopenic purpura. Blood 45:551–562, 1975.
3. Stuart, M. J., and McKenna, R.: Diseases of coagulation: The platelet and vasculature. *In* Nathan, D. G., and Oski, F. A. (eds.): Hematology of Infancy and Childhood. Philadelphia, W. B. Saunders Company, 1981, pp. 1234–1266.
4. McMillan, R.: Chronic idiopathic thrombocytopenia purpura. N Engl J Med 304:1135–1147, 1981.
5. Rywlin, A. M., Hernandez, J. A., Chastain, D. E., et al.: Ceroid histiocytosis of spleen and blood marrow in idiopathic thrombocytopenic purpura (ITP). Blood 37:587–593, 1971.

SELECTIVE MEDULLARY APLASIAS AND HYPOPLASIAS

Red Cell. Pure red cell aplasia is an uncommon disease manifested by anemia with reticulocytopenia in the peripheral blood and a remarkable scarcity or absence of erythroid precursors in the marrow.[1, 2] In striking contrast to the red cell lineage, granulocyte and megakaryocyte populations are normal. Approximately half of the cases occurring in adults have thymomas. This association has suggested the operation of an immune mechanism that may be mediated by suppressor T-lymphocytes directed specifically against the erythroid precursors. Antibodies against the immature red cells and against erythropoietin have been demonstrated in some patients. An occasional case appears to be related to drug therapy, but in most cases no suspected cause or mechanism can be cited.

Congenital hypoplasia anemia of Blackfan and Diamond is usually evident by the age of six months and presents essentially the same blood and marrow features as the noncongenital cases. A defect in which the erythroblast stem cells do not respond to helper T-lymphocytes has been implicated in the congenital form.

Chronic pure red cell aplasia must be distinguished from acute aplastic crises complicating hereditary spherocytosis, sickle cell disease, and other chronic hemolytic anemias.

Granulocyte. Selective granulocyte aplasia of a magnitude comparable to pure red cell aplasia is rare.[3, 4] It occurs in the rare disease reticular dysgenesis with congenital aleukocytosis and in the exceptional case of drug-induced agranulocytosis. Usually granulocyte aplasia occurs as part of generalized medullary aplasia.

Granulocytopenia or neutropenia is more common and is manifested in the marrow either as a hypoplasia of granulocyte precursors at all levels of maturation or as an absence of developmental stages beyond the myelocyte (Figs. 7–7A and B). The latter condition is customarily referred to as maturation arrest. This term is misleading because maturation undoubtedly does occur, but the more mature cells are lost by intramedullary destruction, are sequestered in the marginal granulocyte pool, or have had in-

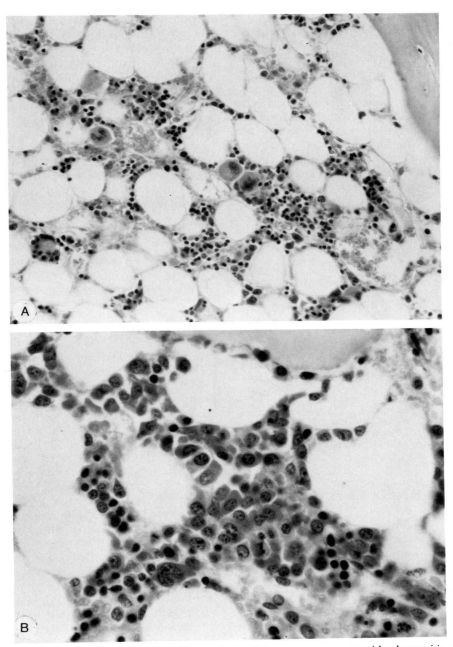

Figure 7–7. A and B. Phenylbutazone-related agranulocytosis in a young woman with pharyngitis, peritonsillar cellulitis, perirectal abscess, and gram-positive septicemia. The moderately cellular marrow contains a normal number of qualitatively normal megakaryocytes and an almost normal complement of late normoblasts but only small scattered clusters of myelocytes. Most remarkable is the striking lack of metamyelocytes and mature neutrophils. The latter finding was reflected in the peripheral blood by a complete absence of circulating neutrophils, either mature or immature. 250× and 520×, H&E.

sufficient time to develop in a marrow that is recovering from chemotherapy or from inadvertent suppression. There is evidence that these mechanisms take place in drug-related neutropenia and in some cases of Felty's syndrome, lupus erythematosis, and similar diseases. Qualitative cytological abnormalities are rarely found in neutropenia except when there is a vitamin B_{12} or folate deficiency.

Megakaryocyte. Selective megakaryocytic aplasia or hypoplasia is rare. More commonly the lack of megakaryocytes is part of a generalized medullary aplasia.[5] In the rare diseases congenital hypoplastic thrombocytopenia with absent radii and megakaryocytic hypoplasia without other somatic defects the lack of megakaryocytes is the sole marrow abnormality. Whether congenital or consequent to radiation, chemical exposure, or therapy, the decrease of megakaryocytes is associated with an increase in megakaryocyte cytoplasmic volume. This is presumably a consequence of a thrombocytopenic stimulus.

REFERENCES

1. Erslev, A. J.: Pure red cell aplasia. _In_ Williams, W. J., Beutler, E., Erslev, A. J., and Lichtman, M. A. (eds.): Hematology. New York, McGraw-Hill, 1983, pp. 409–417.
2. Alter, B. P., Potter, N. U., and Li, F. P.: Classification and aetiology of the aplastic anemias. Clin Haematol 7:431–465, 1978.
3. Finch, S. C.: Neutropenia. _In_ Williams, W. J., Beutler, E., Erslev, A. J., and Lichtman, M. A. (eds.): Hematology. New York, McGraw-Hill, 1983, pp. 773–793.
4. Price, T. H., and Dale, D. C.: The selective neutropenias. Clin Haematol 7:501–521, 1978.
5. Slichter, J. J., and Harker, L. A.: Mechanisms and management of defects in platelet production. Clin Haematol 7:523–539, 1978.

GENERALIZED MEDULLARY APLASIA

The term "aplastic anemia" is traditionally applied to the combination of pronounced anemia, neutropenia, and thrombocytopenia when there is a profound lack of the associated precursor cells in the marrow.[1, 2] Mono- or bicytopenia with a selective lack of only specific precursors or failure in their complete or normal maturation must be distinguished from aplastic anemia because of etiological, therapeutic, and prognostic implications. A more precise terminology currently being introduced is medullary or bone marrow aplasia or hypoplasia, either generalized or selective, with the latter adjective being followed by the cell series involved.

The clinical manifestations of generalized medullary aplasia—pallor, infection, or bleeding, alone or in combination—are consequences of the ensuing pancytopenia. Significant enlargement of the liver, spleen, or lymph nodes is never present.

Core marrow biopsy is a requisite for valid diagnosis. Assessment of marrow cellularity by a smear or section preparation of aspirates is unreliable. The cellularity of the marrow in tissue sections obtained from the iliac crest of a population free of hematological disease has been established according to age-specific groups and serves as a basis for the semi-quantification of diagnostic core specimens.[3] In cases in which the diagnosis of aplasia or hypoplasia is not decisive on the basis of a single core specimen, multiple cores from both iliac crests must be evaluated.

Quantitative evaluation of the marrow core section is deceptively simple, but meticulous qualitative assessment is necessary to avoid confusion with acute leukemia in a phase of marked marrow hypoplasia or with a form of myelodysplasia. Marrow smear preparations may aid cytological evaluation, provided that sufficient numbers of hematopoietic cells are obtained. In generalized medullary aplasia the intertrabecular space is filled almost entirely by mature fat cells (Figs. 7–8 and 7–9). Small numbers of lymphocytes and macrophages are commonly intercalated between the fat cells, with the macrophages frequently being filled with hemosiderin. When present, plasma cells are usually aligned along capillaries. Mast cells cannot be recognized in the standard core sections. Since there may be a few normoblasts, granulocyte precursors, or megakaryocytes, the distinction between generalized medullary aplasia and severe hypoplasia may be arbitrary. Qualitative abnormalities such as megaloblastic maturation or the presence of homogeneous clusters of immature or partially mature cells, however, are indicative of dysplasia or leukemia rather than simply hypoplasia. Serous atrophy of the fat and osteoporosis can be present as manifestations of chronic disease. Focal hemorrhage may occur with biopsy as a result of severe thrombocytopenia. There may be a slight increase in reticulin fibers but not of collagen. Patches of collagen in hypoplastic marrow usually indicate the presence of leukemia or meta-

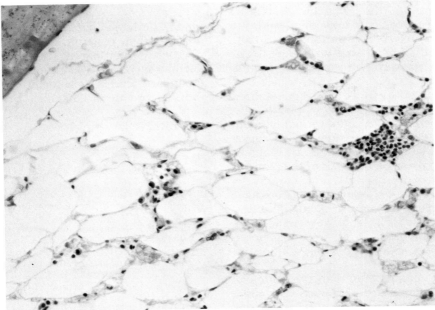

Figure 7–8. Generalized marrow aplasia temporally related to gold and penicillamine therapy for severe rheumatoid arthritis. A few mature lymphocytes and hemosiderin-laden histiocytes are the only remaining hematopoietic occupants of the marrow space, which is otherwise filled by mature fat cells. 250×, H&E.

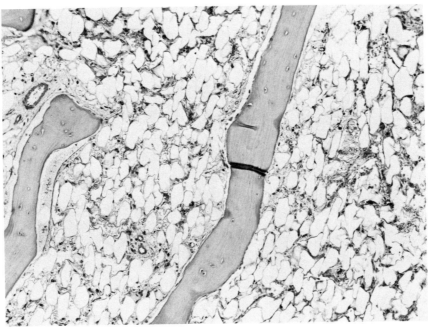

Figure 7–9. Generalized marrow aplasia status 27 days after chemotherapy, total body irradiation, and autologous marrow infusion after relapse in a case of acute myelomonocytic leukemia. There is no evidence of engraftment. 100×, H&E.

static cancer in nearby marrow. When sufficient hematopoiesis fails to occur in the reconstitution of the marrow following chemotherapy for acute leukemia, the histologic results may be indistinguishable from those of medullary aplasia consequent to any other cause. However, this situation is unusual.

The great majority of cases of generalized medullary aplasia are acquired, but in most instances the causative agent cannot be identified. Aplasia or severe hypoplasia consequent to radiation or chemotherapy is almost always recognized on the basis of the patient's history. Infectious hepatitis and mononucleosis are rare causes. Numerous drugs have been suspected as causative, but with few exceptions proof is lacking. Nevertheless, the first therapeutic step in all cases of generalized medullary aplasia is to cease administration of all drugs.

Fanconi's anemia, non-Fanconi's familial aplastic anemia, and dyskeratosis congenita, when they are fully manifest, have marrow pathology indistinguishable from the far more frequent generalized aplasia.

Progression or conversion to acute lymphoblastic leukemia[4] or myeloblastic leukemia occurs in generalized medullary aplasia irrespective of apparent etiology. This potential has served as the rationale for viewing medullary aplasia as a form of dysplasia or the initial phase of leukemia.

REFERENCES

1. Erslev, A. J.: Aplastic anemia. *In* Williams, W. J., Beutler, E., Erslev, A. J., and Lichtman, M. A. (eds.): Hematology. New York, McGraw-Hill, 1983, pp. 151–170.
2. Alter, B. P., Potter, N. U., and Li, F. P.: Classification and aetiology of the aplastic anemias. Clin Haematol 7:431–465, 1978.
3. Hartsock, R. J., Smith, E. B., and Petty, C. S.: Normal variations with aging of the amount of hematopoietic tissue in bone marrow from the anterior iliac crest. Am J Clin Pathol 43:326–331, 1965.
4. Breatnach, F., Chessells, J. M., and Greaves, M. F.: The aplastic presentation of childhood leukaemia: A feature of common-ALL. Br J Haematol 49:387–393, 1981.

MISCELLANEOUS DISEASES

RENAL OSTEODYSTROPHY

Chronic renal failure is attended by complications that can be manifested in both bone and bone marrow. Among these complications are osteodystrophy, anemia, and bleeding.[1, 2] Dialysis has dramatically increased the frequency of the bone disease, has had no effect on the anemia, and has contributed to lessening the occurrence of significant bleeding.

Renal osteodystrophy is produced by a combined destruction and aberrant reconstruction of cortical and trabecular bone. The results are expressed as osteitis fibrosa, osteomalacia, and osteosclerosis. In its mild form, the osteitis fibrosa is focal and manifested by the presence of an occasional trabecula containing a resorption bay (Fig. 8–1) or a tunnel (Fig. 8–2) filled with delicate fibrous stroma and a few osteoclasts or osteoblasts. Peritrabecular fibrosis may also be present. The fibrous tissue is woven rather than orderly lamellar collagen and serves as a matrix for woven bone. Osteoid, which cannot be distinguished from mineralized bone in the standard decalcified histological section, is commonly overabundant. With progression, the

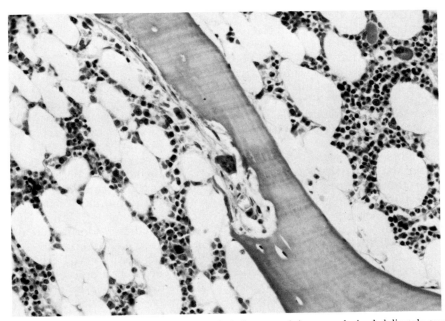

Figure 8–1. The early lesion consists of a small osteolytic bay containing vascularized delicately textured fibrous tissue, an osteoclast, and osteoblasts. Adjacent to the bay, the slightly eroded trabecular surface is covered with osteoblasts. $250 \times$, hematoxylin and eosin stain (H&E).

133

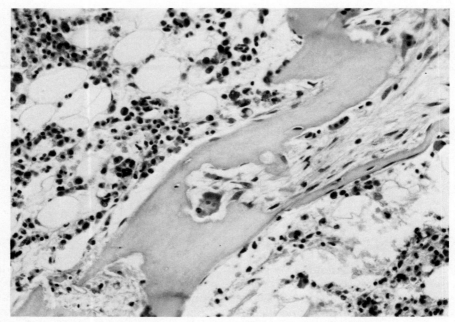

Figure 8–2. The intermediate lesion consists of a trabecular tunnel that is created by osteolysis and filled with finely textured fibrous tissue as the burrowing osteoclasts destroy the bone. 250×, H&E.

lesion becomes widespread, the trabeculae become attenuated and contorted, and the intertrabecular spaces are filled by collagen (Fig. 8–3). Osteoblasts and osteoclasts may partially or totally coat the trabeculae. When osteosclerosis supervenes, thickened and continuous trabeculae of woven bone and osteoid form a dense network and encroach on the marrow space. Although an undecalcified biopsy specimen labeled by tetracycline in vivo is required for maximal evaluation of the bone pathology, most of the features of osteodystrophy are readily identifiable in the decalcified core specimen used for hematological assessment.

The bone pathology of renal osteodystrophy can be simulated by that occurring in primary hyperparathyroidism and thyrotoxicosis. This is especially true in the mild form of the disease when the osteitis fibrosa prevails and the quantity of tissue examined is limited to the standard core specimens (Figs. 8–1 and 8–2). In addition, the more advanced stage can be mimicked by the florid phase of Paget's disease of bone (Figs. 8–3 and 8–4).[3] Currently, in both cases renal disease is the most common cause of this pathology. Osteodystrophy must also be distinguished from the primary hematological diseases that can develop marrow fibrosis and osteosclerosis, and from the fibrosis and bone destruction and bone production induced by metastatic cancer. The morphology of osteoporosis, by contrast, is obviously different (Fig. 8–5).

The status of the marrow is variable. Marked increases in collagen, osteoid, or bone lead to a proportionate displacement of the hematopoietic cells. The cellularity of the residual marrow ranges from very low, consisting primarily of fat cells, to very high. Almost irrespective of the degree of cellularity, erythroid hyperplasia is common. Orthochromatic normoblasts usually predominate, but the number of basophilic forms is increased, reflecting impaired maturation. Commonly hemosiderin increases as a result of impaired iron utilization, hemolysis, and multiple transfusions. There may be megakaryocytic or granulocytic hyperplasia in response to thrombocytopenia or infection, respectively.

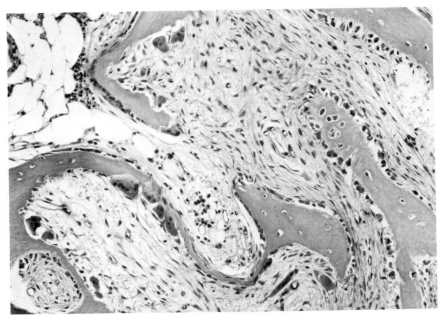

Figure 8–3. The advanced lesion consists of extensive disease with simultaneous osteoclastic bone absorption, osteoblastic woven bone formation, and widespread intertrabecular fibrosis. 170×, H&E.

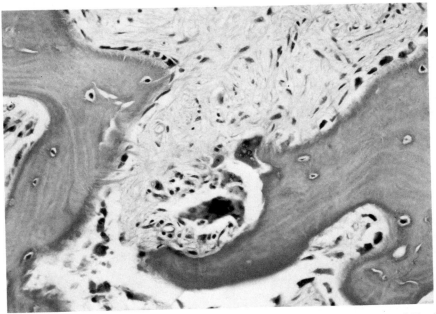

Figure 8–4. Paget's disease of the bone at an intermediate stage in evolution with both lytic and blastic components and abundant fibrous tissue. As a rule the osteoclasts are larger and more highly nucleated than in osteodystrophy. Large thick trabeculae and prominent cement lines are other features that distinguish this disease from osteodystrophy. 250×, H&E.

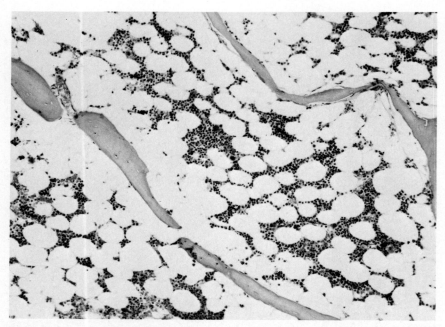

Figure 8–5. Osteoporosis, which is characterized only by attenuated smooth-surfaced trabeculae, has a more dreary morphology when compared with osteodystrophy. 100×, H&E.

REFERENCES

1. Avioli, L. V., and Teitelbaum, S. L.: Renal osteodystrophy. *In* Earley, L. E., and Gottschalk, C. W. (eds.): Strauss and Welt's Diseases of the Kidney. Boston, Little, Brown & Company, 1979, pp. 329–343.
2. Erslev, A. J., and Shapiro, S. S.: Hematologic aspects of renal failure. *In* Earley, L. E., and Gottschalk, C. W. (eds.): Strauss and Welt's Diseases of the Kidney. Boston, Little, Brown & Company, 1979, pp. 277–289.
3. Mirra, J. M.: The skeleton. *In* Coulson, W. F. (ed.): Surgical Pathology. Philadelphia, J. B. Lippincott Company, 1978, pp. 1164–1173.

SEROUS ATROPHY OF MARROW FAT

Pronounced loss of body weight incident to acute or chronic debilitating disease or starvation can be reflected in the marrow fat as well as in the more obvious fat depots. The most common primary diseases associated with serous atrophy of the marrow fat are disseminated cancer, chronic renal disease, malabsorption, and anorexia nervosa.[1] Leukemic marrow following chemotherapy may show focal serous atrophy of the fat during the reconstitution phase.[2] Recognition of the lesion in order that it not be misinterpreted is probably more important than its diagnosis for any therapeutic purpose. It can be misidentified as amyloid and misinterpreted as medullary aplasia, lipoid granulomatosis, or fat necrosis.

The lesion is characterized by a homogeneous extracellular substance separating and surrounding individual fat cells of normal to diminished size. The extracellular material has a very finely fibrillar texture and has been identified as hyaluronic acid (Figs. 8–6 and 8–7). It should be distinguished from fibrin and serum, which can be present in a core specimen as a result of trauma during biopsy.

REFERENCES

1. Seaman, J. P., Kjeldsberg, C. R., and Linder, A.: Gelatinous transformation of the bone marrow. Hum Pathol 9:685–692, 1978.
2. Wittels, B.: Bone marrow biopsy changes following chemotherapy for acute leukemia. Am J Surg Pathol 4:135–142, 1980.

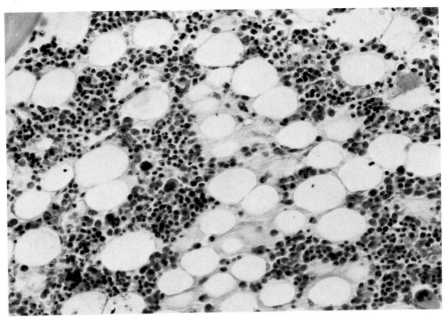

Figure 8–6. Many of the fat cells are partially or totally surrounded by a homogeneous extracellular substance that tends not to intrude among the hematopoietic cells. 250×, H&E.

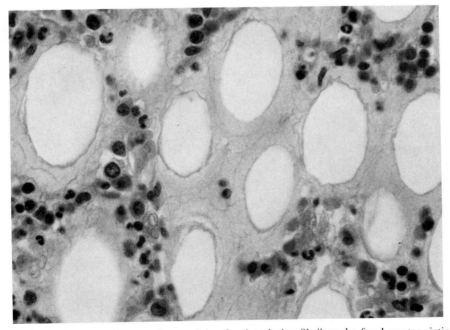

Figure 8–7. The fat cells are set in a matrix containing fine interlacing fibrils and a few hematopoietic cells. 520×, H&E.

BONE MARROW NECROSIS

The diagnostic implications of marrow necrosis are invariably serious. Exclusive of necrotizing inflammatory granulomas, necrotic cells encountered in the marrow space of biopsy core specimens are almost always cancerous and represent metastatic carcinoma or sarcoma, Hodgkin's disease or non-Hodgkin's lymphomas, or leukemia.[1-3] Disorders such as sickle cell disease and caisson's disease, in which bone infarction is the basis of marrow necrosis, are rarely diagnostic considerations at the present time.

The incidence of marrow necrosis is difficult to ascertain. Personal experience is in accord with most published reports and indicates that it is infrequent even in the diseases in which it occurs most commonly. The report of Norgard and coworkers is exceptional in this respect; they report an incidence of approximately 30 per cent in hematopoietic malignancies and in carcinoma metastatic to the marrow.[2] Most of their photographs are difficult to interpret, and their report therefore is difficult to evaluate.

Bone pain appears to be the most frequent symptomatic reflection of marrow necrosis. Anemia with leukoerythrocytosis is the common laboratory finding. This finding, however, is not specific and occurs in leukemia and metastatic carcinoma to the marrow even when there is no necrosis. Among the leukemias, necrosis is most common in the acute lymphoblastic type.[3] There is no evidence that necrosis is related to chemical or radiation therapy. It has been found with equal frequency before and after therapy.

Necrotic cells in the marrow, irrespective of origin or type, have the characteristics displayed by necrotic cells generally: intense eosinophilia when stained with hematoxylin and eosin, amorphous and smudgy cytoplasm, and nuclear pyknosis and fragmentation. The necrosis may be focal or extensive (Fig. 8–8), or there may be a mingling of necrotic and apparently viable cells (Fig. 8–9). Extensive confluent areas of necrotic marrow may be separated from viable areas by a zone laden with neutrophils, that is, by an inflammatory reaction zone. Small pools of densely packed fibrin with entrapped cells should not be confused with foci of necrotic cells. In an occasional case the associated trabecular bone is necrotic, as indicated by the loss of osteocytes. Even in the nonviable state these trabeculae can serve as scaffolds for woven or lamellar bone formation.

The prognostic implication of marrow necrosis in leukemia or lymphoma is not clear.

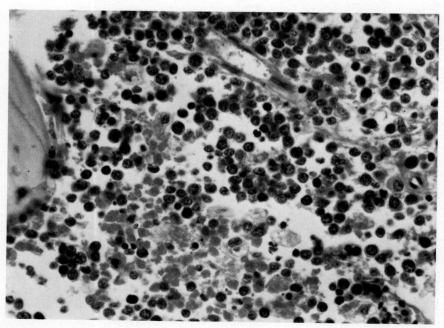

Figure 8–8. Extensive confluent infarction of marrow in Burkitt's lymphoma before chemotherapy. The blast cells are eosinophilic shadows of their viable state. 400×, H&E.

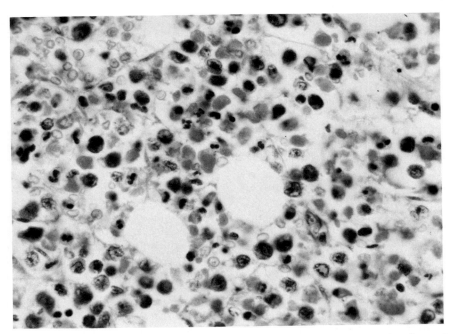

Figure 8–9. Individual cell necrosis in the marrow from a case of acute myeloblastic leukemia prior to chemotherapy. Some of the properly staining cells may be injured, as indicated by their smudgy appearance. 520×, H&E.

There is no evidence that response to therapy is influenced. The development of generalized marrow fibrosis as a consequence of necrosis has been suggested but not proved. This must be distinguished from the localized fibrosis of healing bone infarcts. Necrosis has not been shown to have a role in marrow fibrosis that develops in some cases of leukemia before or after treatment. The suggestion that it plays a role in the development of chronic primary myelofibrosis has no foundation.[4]

REFERENCES

1. Kiraly, J. F. III, and Wheby, M. S.: Bone marrow necrosis. Am J Med 60:361–368, 1976.
2. Norgard, M. J., Carpenter, J. T., and Conrad, M. E.: Bone marrow necrosis and degeneration. Ann Intern Med 139:905–911, 1979.
3. Kundel, D. W., Brecher, G., Bodey, G. P., et al.: Reticulin fibrosis and bone infarction in acute leukemia. Implications for prognosis. Blood 23:526–544, 1964.
4. Conrad, M. E., and Carpenter, J. T.: Bone marrow necrosis. Am J Hematol 7:181–189, 1979.

METASTATIC CANCER

Invasion of the marrow by metastatic cancer occurs primarily, if not solely, by way of the blood stream. The only verifiable exception to the hematogenous route is direct penetration through the cortex by a tumor growing adjacent to a bone. A role for lymphatic channels, if they exist in the marrow, is inconclusive.[1]

The vertebral venous plexus with its variable flow patterns probably serves as the principal conduit to the marrow from the organs that are the most frequent sources of metastatic cancer.[1] This relationship would explain the high frequency of metastases to the vertebral and pelvic bones. In view of this anatomic predilection, the iliac crest has proved to be an efficacious site for biopsy in searching for bone metastases.

Radionuclide bone imaging is a far more sensitive detector of bone metastases than standard bone radiography.[2] This has obviated the need for marrow biopsy as a routine procedure in the clinical staging of carcinoma. Nevertheless, the biopsy may be necessary and can yield definitive information under certain circumstances, including: (1) equivocal results from radionuclide bone imaging; (2) the presence of micrometastases or of large metastases that have no secondary effect on the bone or bone blood flow; and (3) cases in which the morphological features of the metastases can be useful in defining an unknown primary lesion.

Tumor deposits in the marrow commonly provoke fibrosis, bone destruction (osteolysis), or bone formation (osteoplasia) singly or in combination.[1] The osteolysis is rarely associated with the presence of osteoclasts. The osteoplasia results in woven bone, lamellar bone, or mixtures of both. Necrosis of the tumor is common and may be accompanied by necrosis of the fibrous tissue and bone. Unexplained fibrosis and bone changes in a core specimen may be caused by metastatic tumor immediately adjacent to the biopsy site.

The relative efficacies of smears and sections of aspirated marrow particles and of sections of marrow cores from the iliac crest have been investigated and debated.[3–6] While the efficiency of the techniques appears to vary with the primary source of the tumor, the size of the tumor deposit and the degrees of associated fibrosis and bone formation are probably more relevant. False-positive and false-negative results are most likely to be avoided if at least two of the three methods are used. Currently, the combination of smears of aspirated marrow particles and sections of marrow cores appears to be most widely used.

In adults carcinomas of the breast, lung, and prostate account for the majority of metastases encountered in marrow aspirates and core specimens obtained from the iliac crest during diagnostic studies.[4, 7] Less common sources are the gastrointestinal tract, kidney, and skin. From the skin melanomas are the most frequent primary lesion. Sarcomas appear to metastasize to the marrow infrequently despite their predilection for hematogenous dissemination.

In pediatric patients and young adults neuroblastoma, rhabdomyosarcoma, and Ewing's sarcoma constitute the majority of tumors metastasizing to the iliac crest marrow.[7]

The histological and cytological characteristics of the metastatic cancer in combination with the secondary responses are frequently sufficient to predict the type of primary cancer and the source. Accuracy is increased by knowing the age and sex of the patient.

Specific characteristics of the commonly encountered marrow metastases follow.

Lung. Squamous cell carcinoma and adenocarcinoma are more common than small cell anaplastic carcinoma, but the latter type metastasizes more rapidly and frequently than the others (Figs. 8–10 A–F).[8, 9] Based on one series of patients studied before therapy, the frequencies of marrow metastases for these three types are 15, 5, and 20 per cent of cases, respectively.[7] The cytological distinctions of these and of the less frequent large cell type are generally maintained in the marrow deposits, as are those of the small cell carcinoma subtypes. The latter are accompanied by fibroplasia in about 65 per cent of cases and by new bone formation in about 20 per cent.[8, 9] By contrast, in the other types fibroplasia is minimal and an osteoblastic reaction unusual. Evidence of bone destruction is uncommon in all types although it is commonly detected post mortem.

Hansen has reported that in small cell carcinoma aspirates of marrow particles are positive for tumor more frequently than are core specimen sections.[10] While this is not a uniform experience, the use of both methods in each case should yield the best results.

Breast. Unlike carcinomas of the lung, there is no propensity for any histological type of breast carcinoma to metastasize to the marrow more frequently than any other (Figs. 8–11 A–D). Metastases are common, and the pelvic bones are among the sites most frequently affected.[11] In series comprising over 100 cases studied for diagnostic staging, rates up to 28 per cent have been reported.[7, 12, 13]

The most common histological picture in the marrow metastasis is single cells or cells in nests or cords embedded in dense fibrous tissue. A few signet ring cells or more or less well formed glands may be present. New bone formation occurs in about 30 per cent of cases and bone destruction in about 15 per cent, with some cases showing signs of both.

Prostate. Bone metastases are common (Figs. 8–12 A–C). The frequency as determined by staging procedures is exceeded only by that of regional lymph node deposits. This is approximately 40 per cent.[14] Bone metastases occur without lymph node and lymph node without bone. The most commonly affected bones are those of the pelvis and lumbar spine.[15]

Almost all sizable tumor deposits incite a pronounced osteoblastic reaction. In the absence of new bone formation a primary source other than the prostate is highly probable. The new bone may assume the pattern of a dense network of woven bone or of many large discrete or connecting irregular trabeculae. Loss of trabecular bone at the site of metastasis, that is, osteolytic lesions, occurs

Text continued on page 148

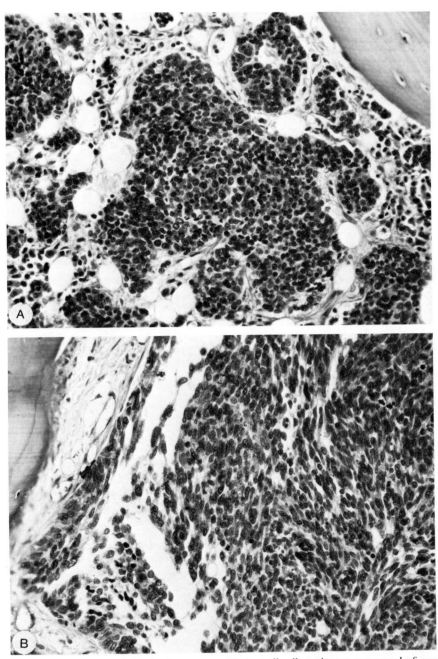

Figure 8–10. Lung carcinoma as evident in the marrow. (*A*) A small cell carcinoma composed of masses of densely packed cells with prominent round nuclei and little cytoplasm. 250×, H&E. (*B*) A small cell carcinoma in which the cells and their nuclei are spindle-shaped. 250×, H&E. (*C*) The focus of a small cell carcinoma, formerly designated as lymphocyte-like, is compared with an aggregate of well-differentiated lymphocytes and intervening hematopoietic cells. 250×, H&E. (*D*) A poorly differentiated squamous cell carcinoma is diagnosed on the basis of more or less distinct intercellular bridges between the polygonal cells. Neither epithelial swirls nor keratin production is present. 250×, H&E. (*E*) This large cell carcinoma with sharply delineated cells is probably a variant of squamous cell carcinoma. 250×, H&E. (*F*) An adenocarcinoma with malformed glands scattered through a fibrous stroma. A shard of infarcted bone is being absorbed by osteoclasts. 250×, H&E.

Illustration continued on following page

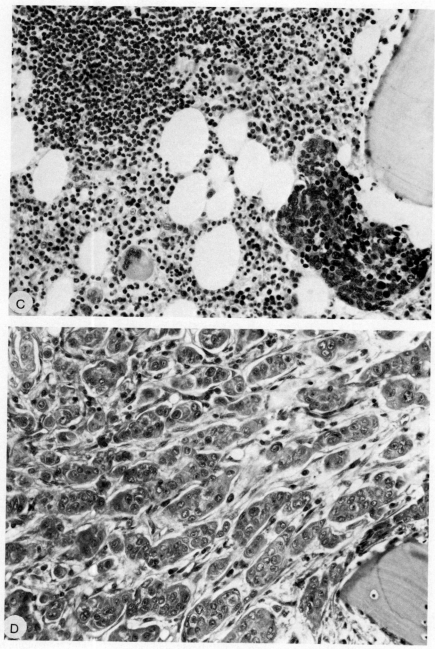

Figure 8–10. *Continued.*

Illustration continued on opposite page

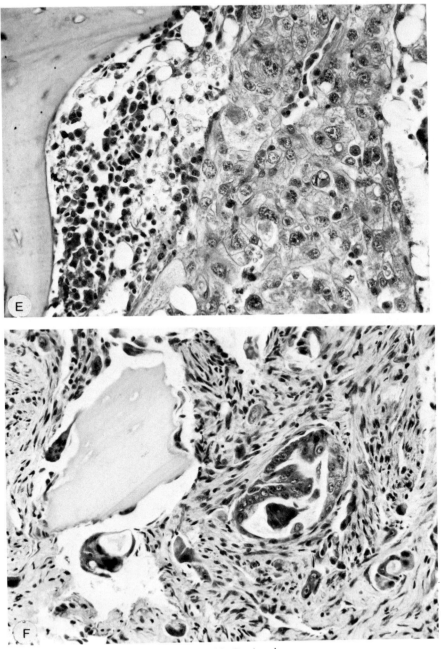

Figure 8–10. *Continued.*

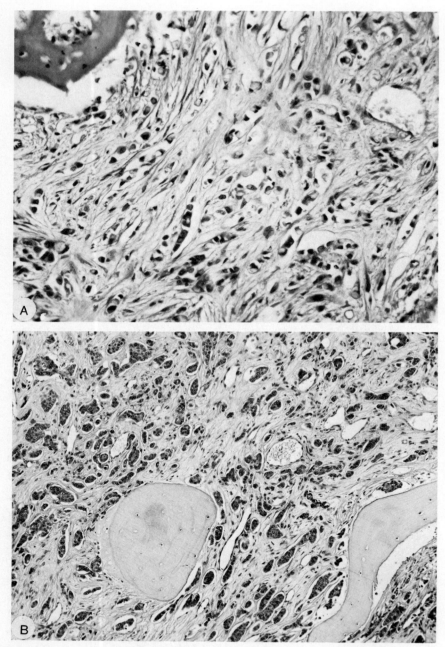

Figure 8–11. Breast carcinoma as evident in the marrow. (*A*) Cancer cells principally as singlets are strewn through a fibrous stoma. Some of the cells contain a cytoplasmic vacuole which is a clue to their adenocarcinomatous nature. 250×, H&E. (*B*) Small clusters of cancer cells are dispersed throughout a fibrous stroma. Since there are no cytogenetic clues beyond the epithelial character of the cells, the lesion is designated as an undifferentiated carcinoma. Woven bone is forming over part of the perimeter of the trabecula in the left lower quadrant. 100×, H&E. (*C*) Both primitive glands and cytoplasmic vacuoles are present in these clusters of cancer cells embedded in dense fibrous stroma. Either the glands or vacuoles are sufficient evidence for the diagnosis of adenocarcinoma. 250×, H&E. (*D*) Unusually well-formed glands are present in this case. There is osteoclast-mediated bone destruction in the left lower quadrant. 250×, H&E.

Illustration continued on opposite page

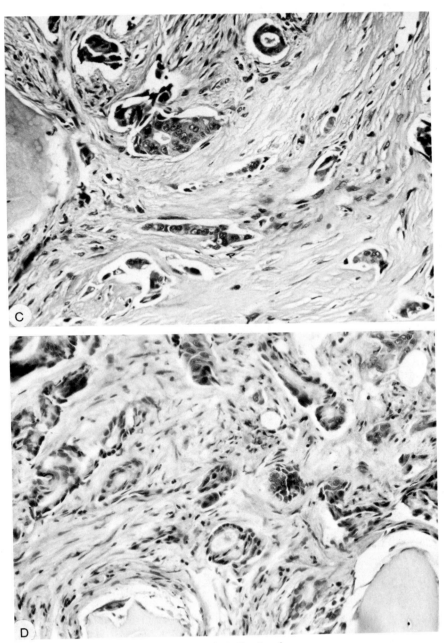

Figure 8–11. *Continued.*

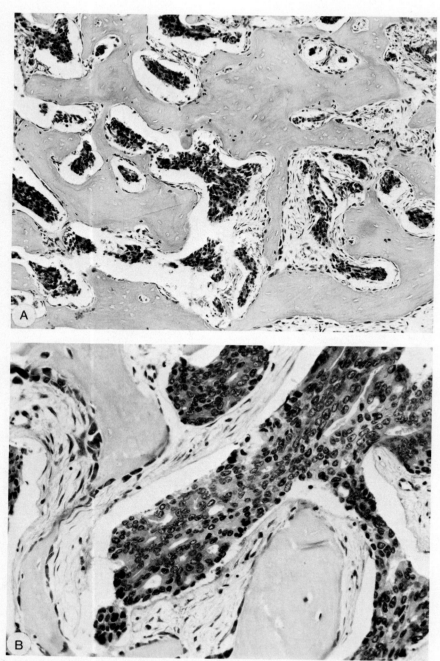

Figure 8–12. Prostate carcinoma as evident in the marrow. (*A*) A striking degree of associated woven bone formation is characteristic of prostate carcinoma deposits. Within the corridors of this maze are the enclaves of cancer cells that are sometimes surrounded by fibrous tissue. 100×, H&E. (*B*) Formation of small glands may be evident in a minority of cases. 250×, H&E. (*C*) Application of the immunoperoxidase technique for the demonstration of prostate-specific antigen or prostatic acid phosphatase can be useful in identifying the prostate as the primary cancer site. 400×, peroxidase antiperoxidase procedure.

Illustration continued on opposite page

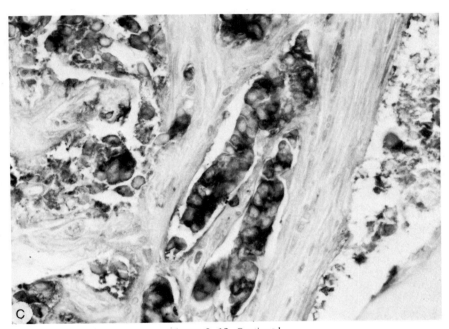

Figure 8–12. *Continued.*

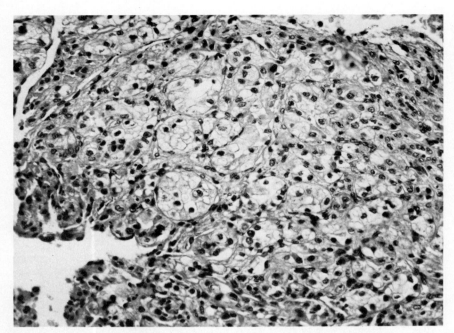

Figure 8–13. Adenocarcinoma of the kidney as evident in the marrow. Presumably derived from renal tubular epithelium, these cancer cells are polygonal, have optically clear cytoplasm around conspicuous nuclei, and cluster into nests. 250×, H&E.

in about 10 per cent of cases. The degree of fibroplasia accompanying the bone reaction is variable. The carcinoma is usually undifferentiated; some degree of gland formation occurs in about 10 per cent of cases.

Less Frequent Tumors. Among the tumors that metastasize to the marrow less frequently and that may display identifiable cytological or histological features are the malignant melanoma and the adenocarcinomas of the kidney, stomach, and colon (Figs. 8–13 to 8–18).[4, 7, 16] Sheets of large polygonal cells

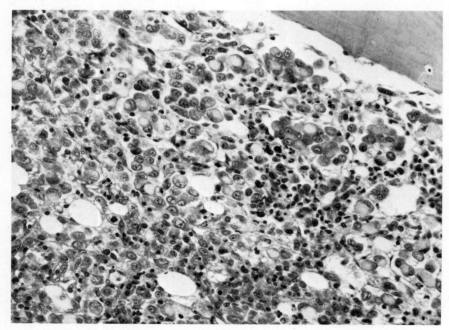

Figure 8–14. Carcinoma of the stomach as evident in the marrow. The presence of a conspicuous cytoplasmic vacuole in many of the cancer cells produces a signet ring configuration. This is common in, but not restricted to, cancers arising in the stomach. 250×, H&E.

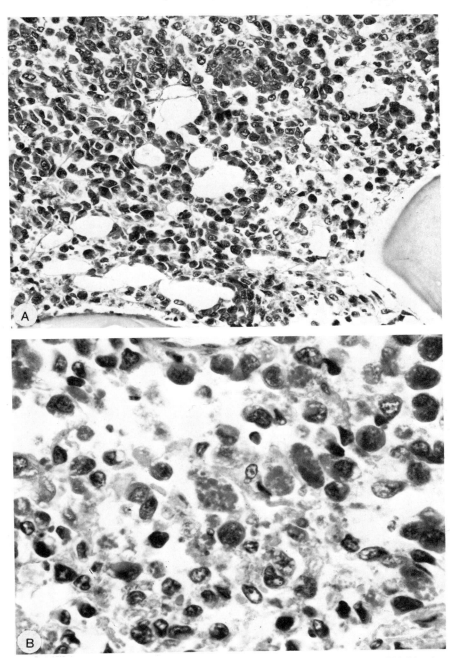

Figure 8–15. Malignant melanoma of the skin as evident in the marrow. In the masses of highly pleomorphic cells, a few contain melanin pigment. This is most evident in the central area at the higher magnification. 250× and 680×, H&E.

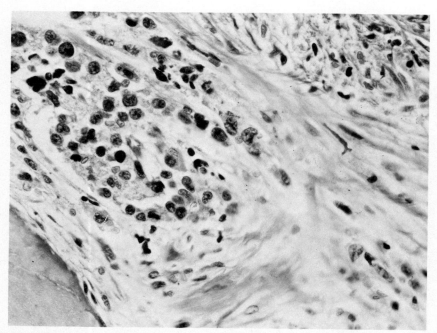

Figure 8–16. Oligodendroglioma of the brain as evident in the marrow. Although cancers originating in the central nervous system rarely metastasize to extraneous locations, surgical operations at the tumor site enhance the likelihood of such metastasis. Two cases of oligodendroglioma arising in the brain and developing marrow metastases postoperatively have occurred at the Duke Hospital. Initially both cases were erroneously diagnosed as myelofibrosis. The deposits are characterized by loosely packed groups of pleomorphic cells gathered in and surrounded by broad bands of fibrous tissue. 400×, H&E.

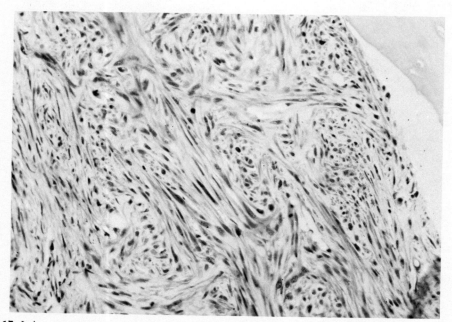

Figure 8–17. Leiomyosarcoma in marrow. Formed by interlacing bundles of myoblasts, this tumor should not be misinterpreted as chronic primary myelofibrosis or simply as fibrosis of the marrow. The high degree of cellularity, the spindle-shaped nuclei, and the mitoses do not occur in reactive fibroplasia. 250×, H&E.

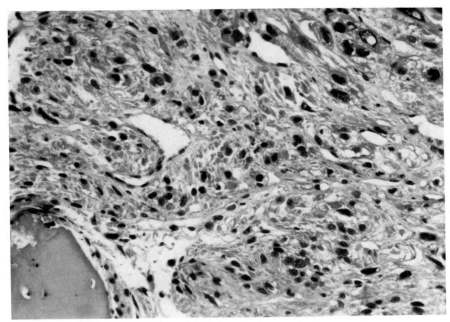

Figure 8–18. Liposarcoma in marrow. Multivacuolated lipoblasts with hyperchromatic pleomorphic nuclei are most evident in the right upper quadrant, but without knowledge of the primary lesion distinction from other malignant soft tissue sarcomas could be difficult. The admonition stated in the legend to Figure 8–17 also applies here. 325×, H&E.

with abundant cytoplasm, which may contain melanin, are characteristic of malignant melanoma deposits in the marrow. When the "hypernephroma" metastasizes as clear cells forming glands, the diagnosis is easily established. Finally, carcinomas arising in the stomach or colon usually disseminate as signet ring cells or cells that form glands.

Mysteriously, nonepithelial cancers in adults rarely implant and grow in the marrow.[7] Over a period of ten years only four such cases have been encountered in the standard core specimens obtained from the iliac crest at the Duke Hospital. These included two cases of oligodendroglioma originating in the brain, a single case of leiomyosarcoma with generalized dissemination but no identified primary site, and one instance of retroperitoneal pleomorphic liposarcoma.

Tumors in Infants and Children. Tumors collectively known colloquially as "cellular blue tumors" or "round cell tumors" pose diagnostic problems when they occur in the marrow just as they may even at their primary site (Figs. 8–19 to 8–21). This group includes neuroblastoma, Ewing's sarcoma, and rhabdomyosarcoma. Distinction from each other and more importantly from acute leukemia and lymphomas is necessary. Certain features that provide useful clues are afforded by sections of core biopsy specimens.

In the neuroblastoma the presence of rosettes with a central meshwork of filamentous fibrils or of cell groups separated by parallel bundles of fibrils is diagnostic. In Ewing's sarcoma the tumor cell nuclei are larger than leukemic blast cells and are more uniform than those in most lymphomas. Furthermore, the sarcoma typically lacks the reticulin network commonly observed in lymphoma. The rhabdomyosarcoma can be identified by its large round, ribbon, or "strap" rhabdomyoblasts scattered among the less differentiated small cells.

The utility of cytochemistry, immunocytology, and electron microscopy in distinguishing between these lesions has been amply publicized.[17–19]

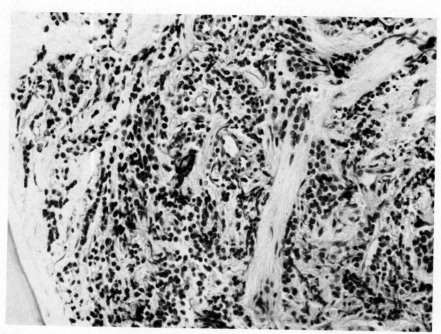

Figure 8–19. Neuroblastoma in marrow. Bundles of fibrils course through masses of cells distinguished only by their small round nuclei. 250×, H&E.

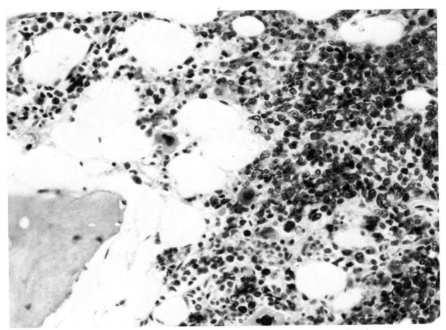

Figure 8–20. Extraskeletal Ewing's sarcoma in marrow. The cells are somewhat larger than those of acute leukemia, but the distinction may be impossible without additional information. 250×, H&E.

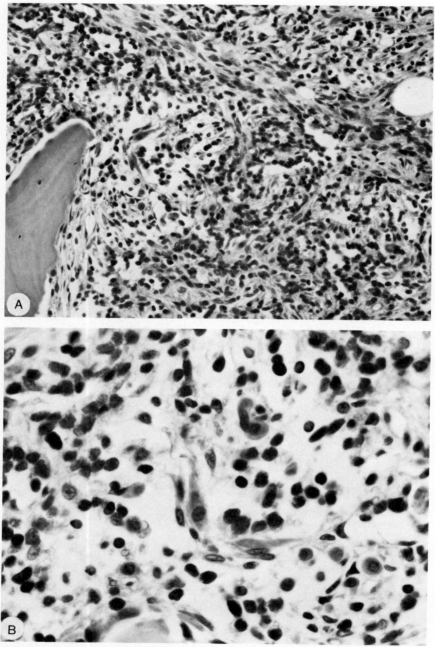

Figure 8–21. Rhabdomyosarcoma in marrow. The presence of ribbon-shaped or giant multinucleated rhabdomyoblasts, most evident at the higher magnification, aids in the identification of this round cell tumor. 250×, 680× and 680×, H&E.

Illustration continued on opposite page

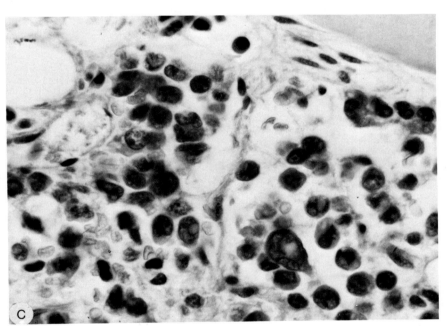

Figure 8–21. *Continued.*

REFERENCES

1. Jaffe, H. L.: Tumors and Tumorous Conditions of the Bones and Joints. Philadelphia, Lea & Febiger, 1961, pp. 589–613.
2. Sugarbaker, P. H., Dunnick, N. R., and Sugarbaker, E. V.: Diagnosis and Staging. *In* DeVita, V. T., Jr., Hellman, S., and Rosenberg, J. A. (eds.): Cancer. Philadelphia, J. B. Lippincott Company, 1982, pp. 233–235.
3. Ellman, L.: Bone marrow biopsy in the evaluation of lymphoma, carcinoma and granulomatous disorders. Am J Med 60:1–7, 1976.
4. Singh, G., Krause, J. R., and Breitfeld, V.: Bone marrow examination for metastatic tumor. Cancer 40:2317–2321, 1977.
5. Savage, R. A., Hoffman, G. C., and Shaker, K.: Diagnostic problems involved in detection of metastatic neoplasms by bone-marrow aspirate compared with needle biopsy. Am J Clin Pathol 70:623–627, 1978.
6. Brynes, R. K., McKenna, R. W., and Sundberg, R. D.: Bone marrow aspiration and trephine biopsy. Am J Clin Pathol 70:753–759, 1978.
7. Anner, R. M., and Drewinko, B.: Frequency and significance of bone marrow involvement by metastatic solid tumors. Cancer 39:1337–1344, 1977.
8. Matthews, M J.: Morphology of lung cancer. Semin Oncol 1:175–182, 1974.
9. Cohen, M. H., and Matthews, M. J.: Small cell bronchogenic carcinoma: A distinct clinicopathologic entity. Semin Oncol 5:234–243, 1978.
10. Hirsch, F., Hansen, H. H., Dombernowsky, P., et al.: Bone-marrow examination in the staging of small-cell anaplastic carcinoma of the lung with special reference to subtyping. Cancer 39: 2563–2567, 1977.
11. Haagensen, G. D.: Diseases of the Breast. Philadelphia, W. B. Saunders Company, 1971, pp. 433–446.
12. Ingle, J. N., Tormey, D. C., and Tan, H. K.: The bone marrow examination in breast cancer. Cancer 41:670–674, 1978.
13. Ridell, B., and Landys, K.: Incidence and histopathology of metastases of mammary carcinoma in biopsies from the posterior iliac crest. Cancer 44:1782–1788, 1979.
14. Catalona, W. J., and Scott, W. W.: Carcinoma of the prostate: A review. J Urol 119:1–8, 1978.
15. Mostofi, F. K., and Price, E. B., Jr.: Tumors of the male genital system. Atlas of Tumor Pathology. Fascicle 8. Washington, D.C., Armed Forces Institute of Pathology, 1973, pp. 232–236.
16. Garrett, T. J., Gee, T. S., Lieberman, P. H., et al.: The role of bone marrow aspiration and biopsy in detecting marrow involvement by nonhematological malignancies. Cancer 38:2401–2403, 1976.
17. Jaffe, N.: Management of malignant solid tumors. *In* Nathan, D. G., and Oski, R. A. (eds.): Hematology of Infancy and Childhood. Philadelphia, W. B. Saunders Company, 1981, pp. 1066–1103.
18. Simone, J. V., Cassady, J. R., and Filler, R. M.: Cancers of childhood. *In* DeVita, V. T., Jr., Hellman, S., and Rosenberg, S. A. (eds.): Cancer. Philadelphia, J. B. Lippincott Company, 1982, pp. 1254–1330.
19. Triche, T. J.: Round cell tumors in childhood: The application of newer techniques to the differential diagnoses. *In* Rosenberg, H. S., and Bernstein, J. (eds.): Perspectives in Pediatric Pathology. Vol. 7. New York, Masson Publishing USA, Inc., 1982, pp. 279–323.

Index

Page numbers in *italics* indicate illustrations; vs. indicates differential diagnosis.

MAJOR PROBLEMS IN PATHOLOGY

MAJOR PROBLEMS IN PATHOLOGY (MPP)—
A series of important monographs focusing on significant topics of current interest. Unsurpassed in clarity and depth of coverage, each hardbound volume in the series is superbly illustrated, and covers a specific issue or disease, a recent advance in clinical therapeutics, or a newly developed diagnostic technique. Each title is written and edited by carefully selected experts of widely recognized ability and authority. In fact, MPP's list of authors is a virtual "Who's Who" of pathology.

Join the MPP Subscriber Plan. You'll receive each new volume in the series upon publication—one to three titles publish each year—and you'll save postage and handling costs! Or you may order MPP titles individually. If not completely satisfied with any volume, you may return it with the invoice within 30 days at no further obligation.

Timely, in-depth coverage you can count on . . . Enroll in the Subscriber Plan for MAJOR PROBLEMS IN PATHOLOGY today!

Available from your bookstore or the publisher.

Complete and Mail Today!

☑ **YES!** Enroll me in the **MAJOR PROBLEMS IN PATHOLOGY** Subscriber Plan so that I may receive future titles in the series immediately upon publication, and save postage and handling costs! If not completely satisfied with any volume, I may return it with the invoice within 30 days at no further obligation.

Name_____

Address_____

City_____State_____Zip_____

☐ Credit my
   salesman

Printed in USA.   283   PM2416E   Postage & handling additional outside USA.

464-3924